THE MIND-BODY
MAKEOVER PROJECT

THE
MIND-BODY
MAKEOVER
PROJECT

A 12-Week Plan for Transforming Your Body and Your Life

Michael Gerrish

Foreword by Cheryl Richardson

Contemporary Books

Chicago   New York   San Francisco   Lisbon   London   Madrid   Mexico City
Milan   New Delhi   San Juan   Seoul   Singapore   Sydney   Toronto

Library of Congress Cataloging-in-Publication Data

Gerrish, Michael.
    The mind-body makeover project : a 12-week plan for transforming your body and your life /
Michael Gerrish; foreword by Cheryl Richardson.
        p.   cm.
    Includes index.
    ISBN 0-07-138250-X (alk. paper)
      1. Health—Case studies.   2. Mind and body—Case studies.   3. Healing—Psychological
aspects—Case studies.   I. Title

RA776.5 G466   2003
613—dc21   2002031564

1 2 3 4 5 6 7 8 9 0 AGM/AGM 1 0 9 8 7 6 5 4 3 2

ISBN 0-07-138250-X

McGraw-Hill books are available at special quantity discounts to use as premiums and sales
promotions, or for use in corporate training programs. For more information, please write to the
Director of Special Sales, Professional Publishing, McGraw-Hill, Two Penn Plaza, New York, NY 10121-
2298. Or contact your local bookstore.

This book is printed on acid-free paper.

To Cheryl

CONTENTS

PART TWO
THE MAKEOVERS

FOREWORD

For years I've listened to people beat themselves up for not eating right or failing to exercise on a consistent basis. As a personal coach and educator I've talked to thousands about their dreams and desires. Time and again when I ask people to identify the one goal that they'd most like to accomplish, the one that would have the greatest impact on their quality of life, the most frequent answer is "I want to lose weight and get in shape!"

If you're reading this Foreword, there's a good chance that you know the frustration and emotional turmoil that come from failed attempts to lose weight and improve your health. You probably feel tortured by a critical inner voice that monitors your eating or exercise habits and reprimands you for breaking yet another promise to yourself when you fail to follow through. And I'm sure that, like so many well-intentioned people, you've listened to many experts and/or read plenty of books, desperately searching for the one thing that will restore your willpower and put you out of your misery. Well, look no more.

In your hands lies the key to freedom—emotional freedom, freedom from the debilitating negative self talk that keeps you caught in a vicious cycle of hope and despair. In this book you'll finally discover the truth about why you haven't been able to lose weight and get in shape, and you'll learn exactly what you need to do to end this cycle once and for all.

When I first considered writing the Foreword for this book, I had a moment of hesitation because the author, Michael Gerrish, is my husband. But as I thought about the millions of people who suffer needlessly with weight and health problems, I knew that it was an important thing for me to do. You see, I know that the process outlined in this book works. For the past ten years I've watched Michael successfully work with individuals just like you who have felt "beaten down" by numerous failed attempts to get in shape. His educational training in both fitness and psychology has given him a knowledge base and perspective that few fitness professionals have. As a result of more than twenty years of experience, Michael has created a process of uncovering and treating a client's unique "unidentified fitness obstacles" (UFOs) which has consistently produced groundbreaking (and lasting) results. This process begins with a one-of-a-kind self diagnostic test. Once you've completed this test, you'll see exactly what stands in your way. Finally, you'll have a clear and accurate picture of the specific personal challenges you're apt to encounter en route to success. You'll see where the bumps in the road will be before they stop you in your tracks.

While developing this test, Michael gave me and several colleagues a chance to try it out for ourselves. All of us were amazed by what came to light as we tallied our scores. When you take the test for yourself, you'll see exactly what I mean. As your obstacles are revealed you'll feel a sense of relief when you discover that it's not your lack of willpower or discipline that's been hindering your success, but rather, problems you weren't aware of or were in denial about. The results of the UFO test will provide you with the all important foundation that is so often missing in most fitness programs. As a matter of fact, I believe this test should be standard procedure for anyone who is considering a diet or exercise program, and an essential tool for any fitness professional who is committed to his or her client's success.

I also know that this program works because I had the privilege of being part of the "makeover team" who worked closely with the seven individuals profiled in this book. Their personal stories will give you a unique and intimate look at why millions of Americans who spend billions of dollars each year on diet and exercise products still can't achieve the level of health they desire.

There are reasons why you can't reach your fitness goals. Real reasons. Reasons that most fitness books and weight loss programs never address. Rather than deal with the symptoms, the program outlined in this book deals with the hidden, underlying source of your problem. As you read the journal entries and ongoing dialogues between Michael and each participant, you'll see that each person had his or her own personal obstacles that had to be addressed before they were able to achieve a measurable level of success. For example, for some getting in shape meant addressing unexpected health concerns like attention deficit disorder, food allergies, or a hormone imbalance. For others, it meant facing the painful experiences that caused them to gain weight in an effort to shield themselves from intimacy or abuse.

In *The Mind-Body Makeover Project* you'll also see that diet and exercise changes are not enough. They must be done in combination with life changes for long-lasting success to occur. Your busy schedule, conflicting beliefs, or discomfort with putting your self-care first all play a role in whether or not you'll achieve your fitness goals. In addition to these life changes, you'll also find that, like the participants in this project, you'll come up against other challenges, the pressure to reach your goals immediately, or the normal fear of whether or not you'll be able to stick with the program once you've reached the level of health you desire. Don't worry. Just turn the page and let Michael's wise and compassionate voice guide you. Believe me, you're in good hands.

It is my sincere hope that *The Mind-Body Makeover Project* marks a new beginning for the fitness industry. A beginning that honors the truth about what it takes to achieve good health. As you read through these pages, you'll begin to see that improving your health is a multifaceted and highly personal process that requires patience, understanding, and, above all, self-acceptance. I wish you the best of luck!

CHERYL RICHARDSON

PREFACE

If you ever want to impress your friends with the volume of mail you receive, put the word out that you're looking for folks who would like makeover for free. Not only would you be amazed by the number of people who'd write (to apply), you would also be deeply moved by their genuine, heartfelt pleas for help. The replies I received, for example, ran from those who had "let themselves go," to those who had serious health concerns and feared they might even *die* (stories like this are what made me regret that I couldn't respond to them *all*). Here are some excerpts from only a few of the letters I received:

> Five years ago, my twenty-month-old son and I survived being struck by a tractor-trailer truck traveling 56 miles per hour. Eight people were killed, including my husband. . . . I have successfully worked through much of my anxiety, depression, survivor's guilt, and post-traumatic stress. However, my body does not reflect the work I've done internally. To me, this is a sign that there is more work to be done.

> Significant milestones in my exercise history include getting rid of the Soloflex (that was in my garage) to make room for the Nordic Track (that was in my house). As my insight expands, so too does my collection of diet books, motivational tapes, health club newsletters, and unfortunately, my waist. I now weigh 19S pounds (leaning 15 degrees to either side of the scale).

> I'm scared that I'll lose my husband because he is obese. He's a warm and loving person who always gives so much. In many ways, he's saved my life— I want to help save his.

> As my husband lay dying, I promised him that I would take better care of myself. But I can't do it alone. To participate in your program just might save my life.

Someday I'd like to get married, or at least find someone to date. But most of my first dates are last dates, and I know it's because of my weight.

I feel like the ceiling of the Sistine Chapel—like this beautiful work of art that's been fading over time, that needs someone to help define my edges, brighten my colors, and let me see again that I am a masterpiece.

What saddened me most of all about these stories, and took me aback, was the fact that just about *everyone* said, "I'm ashamed of the way I look." Quite a few people sent photographs of themselves in loose-fitting clothes, making it hard to accurately assess their size or weight. Others sent photos in which they were just tiny specks in the midst of a crowd, or hiding behind other people, trying their best to avoid being seen. And some letters came without photos, from people who claimed they had nothing to send! Most of them said they were camera shy because they were so overweight and never let anyone photograph them, not even at family events.

Hearing, and seeing, this time and again confirmed an important truth that getting in shape and developing self-esteem is an inside job. It also confirmed the need for a whole new way to achieve these ends, one where our bodies and minds aren't viewed, and treated, as separate things.

It's with great admiration and deep respect for everyone who applied, and also for you, the reader, that my vision takes voice in this book. I hope that it guides and inspires you, and helps you be all you can be.

ACKNOWLEDGMENTS

I would like to thank the following friends and colleagues for their help: Chris and Greg Barnes, Joan Borysenko, Stacy and Dom Brice, Bernie Christopher, Stephen Cluney, Teresa Consentino, Christine Cornelisse, Surya Das, Sharon Day, Michael Demerjian, Max Dilley, Tan Doan, Tim Douglas, Aryn Ekstedt-Cluney, Sue Duggan, Rich and Kathy Fettke, Matthew Goldfain, Fred and Frankie Kamlot, Mark Lawless, Nancy Levin, Carol Look, Gary Mack, Jon Marcus, Lynn McCann, Jenna McCarthy, Annette McClelland, Paul Murphy/D'Angelo, Christiane Northrup, M.D., Linda Novotny, Gam Nguyen, Ania O'Connor, Charles Poliquin, Terry Real, Lynn Robinson, Glenn Rothfeld, M.D., Brother Bob Russell, Edward Shea, Jeff Silva, Howard E. Stone, Jr., M.D., Susan Taylor, Ph.D., Bob Tinnon, Peter Valaskatgis, Gary Watson, Whole Health New England (Gwynne, Stephanie, Kristen, Paul, Teresa), Susan Wormwood, Robin Wunsh, Jon Younger, Ashley Carroll-Whittenberger, Gold's Gym in Salisbury, Mass., and the folks at McGraw-Hill/Contemporary, including Rena Copperman, Mandy Huber, Linda Gorman, Eileen Lamadore, Tom Lau, Marisa L'Heureux, Lynda Luppino, Ann Pryor, Philip Ruppel, and Monica Stoll.

I would also like to thank Nautilus Group, Inc., for the diagrams in Chapter Four, the Lexington Astros baseball team, and publicist Heidi Krupp.

Thanks to my nieces and nephews: Mark, Briana, Grace, Andrew, Christina, Matt, Stephie, David, James, Olivia, J.R., Tommy, John, Liamarie, Lindsay, Justine, Rachel, and Jake. There. Now you can tell your friends that your name is in a book!

Thanks also to my sisters-in-law: Marybeth, Jeanne, Diane, Donna, Lisa, Michelle, Kerri, Missy, Jan, and Karen; my brothers-in-law: Steve, Bob ("Riv"), Tom, Walter, and Mark; my brothers: Tom, Paul, and Chris Gerrish; and my parents-in-law: John and Ann Richardson.

Thanks to Laura Franklin for doing the maintenance on my site. Also, thanks to Shae Inglis and Acro Media, Inc.

Special thanks to artists George Karalias and Peter Beach. Also thanks to The Studio clothing store in Brookline, Mass.

Thanks to my bright, amazingly pleasant editor, Betsy Lane, who somehow managed to help me make the deadline for this book. And a big thanks to Judith McCarthy for taking the reins coming down the home stretch.

Thanks to my agent, John Willig, one of the nicest guys I know. Thanks for all of your great support and guidance over the years.

For their time on the teleclasses, thanks to the Mind-Body Makeover team, especially Cheryl, Debbie Ford, and Tracy Gaudet, M.D. Also thanks to Beth Garland for helping Barry with everyone's hair, and Jonathan Berg, D.C., for being the world's most supportive friend.

This project would not have been possible if it weren't for Ginger Burr, image/skin care consultant, and makeup artist extraordinaire. I can't imagine anyone being as good at what you do.

Kudos to Barry Crites, as well, for the job on everyone's do (I thought about using a Flowbee at first, but luckily, I had you!). You are a hairstyling genius (and a really great person, too).

Also, thanks to Jack Foley for all of the photographs in this book. You are a talented artist and your work is unsurpassed. Thanks for being so flexible, easy to work with, and enthused.

Thanks to "Super" Jan Silva for handling all of the scheduling stuff. There's no one like you when it comes to finding things out and getting things done.

To all of the makeover subjects . . . thank you just for being yourselves. A nicer group of people I could never have hoped to meet. Thanks to Mandy Aronson, L'Tanya Durante, Nina Gibson, Bob Hofeldt, Chet Lyons, Claudia Peresman, and Jennifer Rice. It was a great pleasure to work with you all and I'm sure we'll meet again!

To my parents, Curt and Pat Gerrish, thanks for all that you are, and do. I'm fortunate to have parents who are such big fans of my work.

And last, to my wife, Cheryl Richardson . . . I cannot thank you enough. I don't know anyone who walks her talk as well as you. Thank you so much for inspiring me to always do my best.

INTRODUCTION

This book provides an intimate look at the challenge of getting fit. It will help you to see that when you fail to achieve your physical goals, there are often more than diet or exercise obstacles at the root. It will also help you to see that in order to reach, and *surpass*, your goals, it's important to be more patient and better informed when selecting your paths. I make this point because people are often impulsive when new fads emerge and much too quick to believe in the "miracle" workout or diet du jour. For example, what new ground-breaking trends have captured *your* fancy of late? How many of them are you going to try, and reject, once the novelty fades? How can you trust that you're getting advice that is not going to lead you astray?

What follows are four guidelines that I use as a framework for weighing advice. If what you have read or been told makes sense with regard to the following points, you're probably getting objective advice that you really can use and trust. Here is why you can trust the advice in this book (and what sets it apart).

GUIDELINE #1

This book reveals how people like you have overcome blocks to success. After my first book was published, I received quite a bit of mail. What people were telling me, time and again, was something I took to heart: "I enjoyed the personal stories most, and boy, could I ever relate!" But I also observed a common complaint: "The stories were much too short!" Readers asked to hear more about those I referred to in the book, especially with regard to how they cleared hurdles en route to success. This book will answer their plea by sharing more "trials of the fitness impaired," this time featuring folks who have also been challenged to shape up their *lives*. Over the course of twelve weeks their stories are viewed and discussed in-depth, revealing not only how *they* found success, but how *you* can find it too.

What makes this book different from others (and from the stories in magazines) is the intimate way that it mirrors each person's experience, gainful or not. Instead of just getting a brief, superficial account of how each person fares, you get windows into their minds, and hearts, as their twelve-week adventure unfolds. You're helped to see that getting in shape is rarely a linear process, that even in best-case scenarios some setbacks are bound to occur. By showing you how seven people face their fears, stumbling blocks, and self-doubts, this book provides you with insight into new ways to address yours, too.

While clearly this isn't the only book to feature a plan to get fit, it differs from most by addressing concerns that are often ignored or missed. It differs, as well, by not presupposing that everyone's path is the same and by not showing "after photos" that are retouched or designed to mislead. It's also important to note that most after photos show *best-case* results—results that don't truly reflect what the average person can hope to achieve. Again, this book is unique in that it shows and tells the truth. All of the stories you'll hear, and photos you'll see, are of people like *you*.

GUIDELINE #2

This book challenges common beliefs and provides new ideas to explore. Here are a few examples of ways this book offers new food for thought:

- *Energy Block Acutherapy (EBA)*. Oftentimes, people are faced with blocks that they can't recognize or name. For example, if you're unfocused and thus find it hard to follow a plan, it could be because you have attention deficit disorder, food allergies, or PMS. You might even do self-defeating things without any clue as to why. According to energy therapists (who provide treatment for "energy blocks"), people are prone to self-sabotage when their energy fields are "reversed." With muscle tests to determine if (and how) this applies to *you*, and powerful new techniques that target the root of reversal-based blocks, this book shows you how to rapidly change self-defeating patterns and thoughts. Although there are other terms that are commonly used to describe these techniques, my name for them is energy block acutherapy (EBA). It borrows from popular methods like TFT and EFT (thought field therapy and emotional freedom techniques) to tailor a plan that thwarts your *emotional* blocks to becoming more fit. You'll learn how by "tapping" meridian points and using the right affirmations, you can quickly release any energy blocks that have been sabotaging your gains. You'll also learn targeted treatments that will address very common concerns, for example, to overcome lethargy, cravings, shame, "snack amnesia," or guilt. In essence, you'll see how energy blocks can be fitness and diet blocks, too.

- *Unidentified Fitness Obstacles (UFOs)*. What is the primary reason most of us struggle to get into shape? Experts explain that it's mainly because we're unfocused or uninspired, and the "cure" is to find the right person (or plan) to serve as a coach or guide. Others claim that it's simply a matter of learning to toughen up. "Pull yourself up by the bootstraps" or "Just do it," as Nike suggests. Easier said than done, I say, and I'm betting that you would agree. Statements like these just make you feel weak and insinuate that you're at fault! You're not inherently lazy, nor are you lacking the will to succeed! The way I see it, laziness is a "symptom," NOT a cause! The *cause* is an "unidentified fitness obstacle" (UFO). UFOs are the hidden blocks that prevent you from reaching your goals, for example, hormone imbalances, shadow beliefs, or chronic fatigue. These are the kinds of things this book will help you expose and address. You'll see why your good intentions keep paving roads that turn into dead ends.

- *The Mind-Body Makeover Team*. In keeping with the theme of this book (holistic transformation), I enlisted a team to offer advice and support as the project progressed. Included were Cheryl Richardson, Tracy Gaudet, and Debbie Ford, as well as other experts who are leaders in various fields. As you follow the makeover stories, noting the path each participant takes, think about how the advice that each person received from the team could help *you*. As you see how the makeover process evolves and hidden blocks come to the fore, you'll learn how to tap the right resource and make better choices when looking for help.

GUIDELINE #3

Instead of just giving you standard advice about how to work out or lose weight, this book speaks to the fact that you also must look at the way you *live*. No diet or exercise program, no matter how great it may be, will ever do much to help you get fit if your life has been out of control. For example, if you've been working too much or your marriage is not on good terms, the stress will drain your energy, leaving you little for anything else. I know that this may sound obvious, but believe me, too often it's not! The things in your life that distract you, or that frequently cause you stress, can affect how much time and attention you give to practicing good self-care, including making a point to eat right or taking the time to work out!

As you read this book, you'll discover why being "selfish" makes good sense. You'll see that by taking more time for yourself—for example, to go to the gym—you'll actually get more done at home and become more productive at work. And you'll see how you can't help *anyone* much if you don't learn to help *yourself* first.

GUIDELINE #4

This book doesn't knock other experts or other approaches to finding success. Putting down peers is a favorite pastime of personal trainers these days, and given that egos are often involved, this doesn't come as a surprise. The way this plays out can vary, but the result is often the same: People keep getting confused about who they should trust and what to believe.

Whenever I'm being given advice about training, or anything else, if I sense that it's biased or ego-induced, I question what I'm being told. Conversely, if I'm getting advice from someone who's gracious and fair, I'm more apt to take it seriously and less apt to put up my guard. A little humility goes a long way when it comes to gaining my trust. And the truth is that there are many paths to getting and staying in shape. The challenge lies in finding the one that is going to be best for *you*.

In summary, Part One of this book provides a plan to make over *yourself*. You'll see how by conquering UFOs (unidentified fitness obstacles), you'll achieve your goals in much less time and reach new heights of success. You'll also learn how to treat energy blocks that are acting as hidden constraints and where you can find the help you'll need to address your specific concerns. Lastly, you're given a simple plan you can use at most any gym, as well as nutritional guidelines you can adapt to your personal needs.

Also in Part One, you'll take a self-diagnostic test. This test will help you to, first, reveal your most prominent UFOs, and second, become more clear about what course of action will serve you best. Then you'll be told what steps to take first and what to expect when you start. As you follow each step, don't be concerned about doing a "perfect" job (there's no perfect way to get into shape, lose weight, or improve your life!). It's even okay if you miss some steps or happen to jumble them up. Once you get the ball rolling, you can retrace them later on.

Part Two shows how seven people (who followed the plan outlined in Part One) fared during the makeover process, each step of the way, from beginning to end. You'll see how as they uncovered their hidden blocks to getting in shape, they gained the self-confidence, knowledge, momentum, and focus required to succeed.

And finally, as opposed to books that are solely about working out, this one examines image and lifestyle concerns, and emotional health. Integrating these areas is the key to holistic health, a state that is best achieved when one seeks change from the *inside* out. Keep in mind as you read this book and apply all the things that you learn that your final goal should be to feel and *live* as well as you *look*. So, let's get your makeover started now! Enjoy the ride and good luck!

TOP TEN ESSENTIAL TIPS FOR MAKING OVER YOUR BODY (AND LIFE)

1. *Expect to fail a number of times before you achieve success.* Cut yourself slack whenever you can and don't dwell so much on your faults. Focus on doing the best you can and getting back up when you fall. Remember that an occasional slip is par for any course.

2. *Learn to trust your instincts and don't judge (or ignore) your moods.* Tune into your feelings more regularly and don't judge yourself when you do. Don't feel compelled to shake feelings off; instead, heed the message they give. Let them act as a guide for determining how and when to shift gears.

3. *As long as you stay objective, it won't hurt to try new things.* Don't make yourself your own guinea pig, though, without asking questions first. For example, find out if the option you want to explore has been used with success, preferably by those who have had very similar goals and concerns. Record what you do each step of the way (in a journal or training log). Remember, if something feels off to you, stop and then reassess your approach.

4. *Stay focused on what success means to YOU; forget about what others think.* Don't use societal standards as a basis for setting your goals. You'll set yourself up to feel like you've failed regardless of what you achieve. Imagine how you would look and feel if you were to be at your best. Is it different from how you *think* you should look or the image you have as a goal?

5. *Learn from what you see others do, but remember that you are unique.* Resist the urge to compete and compare—it'll just send you down the wrong path. Try to keep things in perspective, i.e., we don't all get dealt the same cards. Learn how to play with the hand you've received. Play *well* with the cards you have.

6. *Resist the urge to set lofty goals you'll be slow (or unlikely) to reach.* Instead, be more modest and set "mini-goals" you can reach in a few days or weeks. Achieving success breeds *more* success—it ensures that your efforts are fueled. The longer you have to wait to succeed, the less apt you are to persist.

7. *Stop to celebrate* every *success before you set any more goals.* If you have a habit of raising the bar every time you achieve a goal, you might want to break this pattern by taking more time to savor your feats. You need to acknowledge how far you've *come* to increase how far you'll *go*.

8. *Stop criticizing your body.* It hears everything you think. Think about what you say to yourself and the words that you typically choose. Are they mostly self-defeating words, for example, "I'm not" or "I can't"? Replace all negative statements and thoughts with ones like "I am" and "I can."

9. *If you follow health advice blindly, you'll be sure to run into a wall.* Always consider the source when anyone offers you new advice. Has he or she had success helping those with similar goals (and blocks)?

10. *You're going to fall off your horse now and then, so prepare to keep climbing back on.* Everyone goes off their diet and misses a workout once in a while, but if you climb "back on your horse" when you do, over time you will stop falling off. And, if you find that you're *still* falling off, don't think that you're destined to fail. With patience and practice you'll learn how to center yourself and control the reins.

THE MIND-BODY MAKEOVER PROJECT

PART ONE

The Program

CHAPTER ONE

UNIDENTIFIED FITNESS OBSTACLES

Don't water your weeds.
HARVEY MACKAY

Do you watch what you eat, but the scale won't budge and you don't have a clue as to why? Would you like to exercise more than you do but can't seem to find the time? Perhaps you *are* training regularly and *still* falling short of your goals? If this is the case, there's probably more to the story than you are aware. This chapter will give you new insight into what the real story could be.

More often than not, when the course of action you take to get fit doesn't work, the remedy offered by experts is a new diet or way to work out. The problem with this is that most of the time the big picture gets ignored, and as a result, most people are lucky to find any answers at all. And if they continue this cycle, it's unlikely that they ever will, because the nutrition and exercise part of the puzzle is *only one piece*. The truth is that this puzzle consists of a whole lot of other parts, too, parts that most people misunderstand, are oblivious to, or ignore. I call these other parts, or missing pieces, "UFOs" (unidentified fitness obstacles).

If you're like most folks, and you're struggling to stay on a diet or skipping the gym, the way to turn failure into success is to conquer your UFOs. As opposed to what most fitness experts would say (with regard to what gets in our way), I believe overcoming our UFOs is the key to achieving good health. What also distinguishes my point of view from that of most experts I know is the range and type of issues I cite as barriers to getting fit. For example, though most people know that they need to sleep well to achieve good health, they don't realize the extent to which not sleeping well can restrict their success. Moreover, it's not just insomnia that could act as a UFO; it could be things like sleep apnea or a sleep phase that's advanced or delayed.

This is one of the most important chapters in this book. It will help you to see what *really* is foiling your efforts to get in shape. Once you've completed the following test, what you need to address will be clear.

UFO TEST

Consider the numbers under each statement for each UFO and circle the one that reflects how much you agree or disagree. (If this book is from a library, use a notebook to record your results.)

Rating Scale
1–Strongly Disagree
2–Mostly Disagree
3–Neither Agree nor Disagree
4–Mostly Agree
5–Strongly Agree

UFO I
1. I have random bouts of anxiety (when stress is not clearly the cause).

    1   2   3   4   5

2. I often have blood sugar swings during which I feel restless, then fatigued.

    1   2   3   4   5

3. I often find it hard to wake up and/or get out of bed.

    1   2   3   4   5

4. I'm often startled by people or noise (or I hardly react at all).

    1   2   3   4   5

5. I often feel sluggish or restless—either I'm tired or I can't relax.

    1   2   3   4   5

6. Sometimes I feel like I'm running on fumes (I can barely get through the day).

    1   2   3   4   5

UFO 2

1. Even in warm environments, there are times when I feel cold.

   1   2   3   4   5

2. I often crave sweets and sugary foods, especially when I'm stressed.

   1   2   3   4   5

3. I'm often bothered by allergens, such as mold or chemical fumes.

   1   2   3   4   5

4. Lately I've found it harder to stay on a diet and lose weight.

   1   2   3   4   5

5. More often than not, I feel stressed, unsettled, wired, fatigued, or depressed.

   1   2   3   4   5

6. Lately I've lost some muscle mass or observed that my skin has thinned.

   1   2   3   4   5

UFO 3

1. For the past six months (or longer), I've had less interest in sex.

   1   2   3   4   5

2. For the past six months (or longer), I've been getting a lot less sleep.

   1   2   3   4   5

3. Lately I've lost some body hair and my muscle mass has decreased.

   1   2   3   4   5

4. For the past six months (or longer), I've been irritable and depressed.

   1   2   3   4   5

5. I seem to have gained a lot of fat in the area of my chest.

   1   2   3   4   5

6. I no longer have strong erections (or it's difficult to get aroused).

   1   2   3   4   5

UFO 4 (Women Only)

1. For no apparent reason, I've been gradually gaining weight.

   1   2   3   4   5

2. In the past, I've had uterine fibroids, bladder infections, or night sweats.

   1   2   3   4   5

3. Lately, when I've been premenstrual, my symptoms have been more severe.

   1   2   3   4   5

4. I've been having hot flashes, headaches, and palpitations for three or more months.

   1   2   3   4   5

5. Most of the fat I've gained has been on my hips and upper thighs.

   1   2   3   4   5

6. For at least three months, I've been weepy, bloated, irritable, or fatigued.

   1   2   3   4   5

UFO 5

1. My lower abdominal area is where I'm storing most of my fat.

   1   2   3   4   5

2. Lately I've found that certain foods consistently make me sick.

   1   2   3   4   5

3. Lately I've been more sensitive to toxins and chemical fumes.

   1   2   3   4   5

4. I often feel bloated after a meal and eat even when I feel full.

   1   2   3   4   5

5. My energy level is usually low, especially after a meal.

   1   2   3   4   5

6. I frequently have skin rashes, memory lapses, or diarrhea.

   1   2   3   4   5

UFO 6

1. I have acne, psoriasis, eczema, and/or white spots on my nails.

    1   2   3   4   5

2. I'm frequently very hungry, even at times when my stomach is full.

    1   2   3   4   5

3. I often feel tired and bloated very soon after I finish a meal.

    1   2   3   4   5

4. Throughout the day, I often have an excessive amount of gas.

    1   2   3   4   5

5. Sometimes when I take supplements, I begin to feel nauseous or sick.

    1   2   3   4   5

6. Oftentimes, undigested food is visible in my stools.

    1   2   3   4   5

UFO 7

1. I often feel ill when it's muggy or damp (or I'm around dust or mold).

    1   2   3   4   5

2. I often crave alcohol, sugar, bread, and products containing yeast.

    1   2   3   4   5

3. I often have headaches (with tingling), dizzy or light-headed spells, and "brain fog."

    1   2   3   4   5

4. My skin is often very dry and my hands and feet are cold.

    1   2   3   4   5

5. I often suffer from allergies, colds, urinary infections, or stress.

    1   2   3   4   5

6. Sometimes, first thing in the morning, there is a white coating on my tongue.

    1   2   3   4   5

UFO 8

1. I often feel tired and sluggish and most of my movements are very slow.

   1   2   3   4   5

2. I'm often fatigued in the morning (and it takes me a while to get up).

   1   2   3   4   5

3. My hands and feet are often cold and my temperature tends to be low.

   1   2   3   4   5

4. Even though I work out and watch what I eat, I can't lose weight.

   1   2   3   4   5

5. My skin is dry and pale and/or my hair is dry and coarse.

   1   2   3   4   5

6. Lately I've had menstrual problems or been less interested in sex.

   1   2   3   4   5

UFO 9

1. In the fall and winter, I'm always more depressed, overwhelmed, and fatigued.

   1   2   3   4   5

2. In the fall and winter, I find that I often crave starchy or sugary foods.

   1   2   3   4   5

3. I always feel quite a bit better during the spring and summer months.

   1   2   3   4   5

4. In the fall and winter I sleep a lot more (and spend more time at home).

   1   2   3   4   5

5. I often gain at least 10 pounds in the fall and winter months.

   1   2   3   4   5

6. I always have more energy, and feel better, on sunny days.

   1   2   3   4   5

UFO 10

1. The week before my cycle, I get irritable and tense.

    1   2   3   4   5

2. The week before my cycle, I get bloated (or gain weight).

    1   2   3   4   5

3. Before my cycle, I often feel sluggish, weak, or extremely fatigued.

    1   2   3   4   5

4. I'm more depressed than usual for a week or two each month.

    1   2   3   4   5

5. My cravings increase dramatically for a week or two each month.

    1   2   3   4   5

6. I'm often unfocused and clumsy for a week or two each month.

    1   2   3   4   5

UFO 11

1. I tend to get bored very easily, and often leave tasks half done.

    1   2   3   4   5

2. Pursuing a goal inspires me, but achieving one leaves me "flat."

    1   2   3   4   5

3. I speak or act impulsively and don't often have much tact.

    1   2   3   4   5

4. I'm usually either distracted or I totally tune things out.

    1   2   3   4   5

5. I'm intelligent and creative, but I sabotage my success.

    1   2   3   4   5

6. I crave stimulating activities, but nothing excites me for long.

    1   2   3   4   5

UFO 12

1. At times I binge (compulsively) and force myself to purge.

       1   2   3   4   5

2. I've tried using laxatives, diet pills, or diuretics to lose weight.

       1   2   3   4   5

3. My weight is very unstable (I can gain or lose lots of weight fast).

       1   2   3   4   5

4. I've noticed deterioration of the enamel on my teeth.

       1   2   3   4   5

5. I admit that I have a problem, but it's one that I can't control.

       1   2   3   4   5

6. My stomach and throat are often sore and at times I have swollen glands.

       1   2   3   4   5

UFO 13

1. My weight is 10 or more pounds below the norm for my height and frame.

       1   2   3   4   5

2. I starve myself or eat much less than I need to maintain good health.

       1   2   3   4   5

3. I often get anxious and irritable unless I work out every day.

       1   2   3   4   5

4. I always feel cold, rarely sleep well, and often have very dry skin.

       1   2   3   4   5

5. People have said I'm much too thin and are worried about my health.

       1   2   3   4   5

6. I haven't had a period for several consecutive months.

    1   2   3   4   5

UFO 14

1. I hate certain parts of my body, even though others say I look fine.

    1   2   3   4   5

2. When I look at myself in the mirror, I often see numerous flaws.

    1   2   3   4   5

3. I would like to have plastic surgery on certain parts of my body
   and face.

    1   2   3   4   5

4. There are certain parts of my body that I frequently measure or touch.

    1   2   3   4   5

5. I often need to be reassured about the way I look; for example,
   I doubt that I'm really as thin or as big as everyone thinks.

    1   2   3   4   5

6. I often avoid social settings and wear clothes that hide my "flaws."

    1   2   3   4   5

UFO 15

1. I've been feeling anxious or hopeless, more often than not, for at least
   six months.

    1   2   3   4   5

2. I've been sleeping too much (or too little), more often than not, for at
   least six months.

    1   2   3   4   5

3. For the past six months (or longer), everyday tasks have seemed like
   a chore.

    1   2   3   4   5

4. For at least six months, more often than not, I've been irritable and tense.

    1   2   3   4   5

5. I've been very indecisive, more often than not, for at least six months.

    1   2   3   4   5

6. For at least six months, more often than not, I've suffered from low self-esteem.

    1   2   3   4   5

UFO 16

1. When I eat certain foods, I feel light-headed, faint, congested, or short of breath.

    1   2   3   4   5

2. I frequently notice swelling around my eyes, lips, throat, and tongue.

    1   2   3   4   5

3. I often suffer from acne, eczema, rashes, itching, or hives.

    1   2   3   4   5

4. Oftentimes after eating I feel bloated or full of gas.

    1   2   3   4   5

5. Frequently after eating I get sick or have diarrhea.

    1   2   3   4   5

6. The foods that tend to bother me most are usually those I crave.

    1   2   3   4   5

UFO 17

1. I've noticed that there are certain foods that *often* give me cramps.

    1   2   3   4   5

2. I've noticed that there are certain foods that *always* give me gas.

    1   2   3   4   5

3. There are certain foods that *always* make me bloated or fatigued.

    1   2   3   4   5

4. I've found that certain foods, more often than not, cause diarrhea.

    1   2   3   4   5

5. Certain foods make me queasy, but they're extremely hard to resist.

    1   2   3   4   5

6. The foods that tend to bother me most are usually those I crave.

    1   2   3   4   5

UFO 18

1. I'm sensitive to tobacco smoke, perfumes, and chemical fumes.

    1   2   3   4   5

2. Sometimes I notice itching on the roof of my mouth and throat.

    1   2   3   4   5

3. I'm often able to smell things that other people can't.

    1   2   3   4   5

4. When I clean my house (or have it cleaned), I often feel drained or sick.

    1   2   3   4   5

5. Usually after an hour at work I want to lie down and rest.

    1   2   3   4   5

6. I often feel sick in traffic or become dizzy when smelling paint.

    1   2   3   4   5

UFO 19

1. I've noticed that I sneeze much more at certain times of the year.

    1   2   3   4   5

2. I tend to have itchy or watery eyes at certain times of the year.

    1   2   3   4   5

3. My nose often runs or gets stuffy at a particular time each year.

    1   2   3   4   5

4. I tend to get sinus infections at particular times of the year.

    1   2   3   4   5

5. I often get ear infections at the same time every year.

    1   2   3   4   5

6. I get respiratory infections at around the same time every year.

    1   2   3   4   5

UFO 20

1. When I spend lots of time on my cell phone or near computers, my face becomes flushed, and sometimes my skin begins to itch or I start to develop a rash.

    1   2   3   4   5

2. I often suffer from headaches, light-headed spells, or a tingly scalp.

    1   2   3   4   5

3. I work or live near high-power lines, transformers, or power plants.

    1   2   3   4   5

4. I use a computer, microwave oven, or cell phone almost every day.

    1   2   3   4   5

5. I often can't sleep when I use my computer prior to going to bed.

    1   2   3   4   5

6. Lately I've been less focused and have experienced memory loss.

    1   2   3   4   5

UFO 21

1. Rather than focus on what I *can* do, I focus on what I *can't*.

    1   2   3   4   5

2. I often mix up words when I speak and tend to write letters "reversed."

      1   2   3   4   5

3. It seems like I have a tendency to sabotage my success.

      1   2   3   4   5

4. I know what I want and need to do but often feel hopelessly stuck.

      1   2   3   4   5

5. The harder I try to change myself, the harder it is to change.

      1   2   3   4   5

6. More often than not, I ignore advice and keep heading down the wrong paths.

      1   2   3   4   5

UFO 22

1. I often find it difficult to set boundaries and say no.

      1   2   3   4   5

2. I'd rather make myself suffer than cause pain to someone else.

      1   2   3   4   5

3. I'm susceptible to being bullied, manipulated, or played for a fool.

      1   2   3   4   5

4. I tend to avoid confrontation (I get anxious when conflict occurs).

      1   2   3   4   5

5. I rarely speak up when I'm criticized, hurt, insulted, berated, or blamed.

      1   2   3   4   5

6. When people "talk my head off," I will seldom interrupt.

      1   2   3   4   5

UFO 23

1. I think I'm genetically predisposed to always be overweight.

     1   2   3   4   5

2. I'm lazy and don't have the discipline to pursue important goals.

     1   2   3   4   5

3. When I overeat or my diet is poor, I'll often say that I've been *bad*.

     1   2   3   4   5

4. I'm too busy, clumsy, unfocused, or old to ever get into good shape.

     1   2   3   4   5

5. I avoid working out at a gym, outdoors, or anywhere I can be seen.

     1   2   3   4   5

6. I'm different from other people—my personal problems are unique.

     1   2   3   4   5

UFO 24

1. Because I didn't like gym class, I'll never enjoy working out.

     1   2   3   4   5

2. In gym class, when they were choosing sides, I often was chosen last.

     1   2   3   4   5

3. Working out is boring, vain, uncomfortable, or a chore.

     1   2   3   4   5

4. I avoid working out at a gym, outdoors, or anywhere I can be seen.

     1   2   3   4   5

5. In the past, I often was clumsy (or hurt myself) when I worked out.

     1   2   3   4   5

6. I can't think of any exercise or activity I would enjoy.

     1   2   3   4   5

1. People I know have often tried to sabotage my success.

    1   2   3   4   5

2. I'd exercise more if my spouse/partner/coworker/friend wouldn't put me down.

    1   2   3   4   5

3. Nothing ever works for me—I often expect to fail.

    1   2   3   4   5

4. I'm overweight due to my genes and circumstances beyond my control.

    1   2   3   4   5

5. Because I'm compelled to help others, I don't very often have time for myself.

    1   2   3   4   5

6. I often blame people for doing things that are harmful to my health.

    1   2   3   4   5

UFO 26

1. I don't know how to position myself when using weights or machines.

    1   2   3   4   5

2. I often shrug my shoulders, tense my neck, or arch my back.

    1   2   3   4   5

3. I often use fast, jerky movements that have injured my muscles and joints.

    1   2   3   4   5

4. When performing aerobic exercise, I put a lot of stress on my joints.

    1   2   3   4   5

5. I don't know the best range of motion to use when using weights or machines.

    1   2   3   4   5

6. I seldom feel an exercise (much) in the area I want to work.

    1   2   3   4   5

UFO 27

1. Lately I'm working out harder (and more) but find I keep getting sick.

    1   2   3   4   5

2. Before I begin my workout, most of the time I'm in a bad mood.

    1   2   3   4   5

3. I seldom look forward to working out (it usually feels like a chore).

    1   2   3   4   5

4. I train for ninety minutes or more, sometimes more than three days a week.

    1   2   3   4   5

5. I won't ease up or take time off when I'm injured or fatigued.

    1   2   3   4   5

6. Lately I've noticed I need more time to recover between routines.

    1   2   3   4   5

UFO 28

1. I rarely do more than two aerobic workouts every week.

    1   2   3   4   5

2. I rarely do more than one machine or weight training workout per week.

    1   2   3   4   5

3. I stick to a preplanned number of reps, even though I can often do more.

    1   2   3   4   5

4. I rarely increase my intensity or do anything new when I train.

    1   2   3   4   5

5. I'm afraid to use heavier weights because I fear that I'll get too big.

    1   2   3   4   5

6. I usually go through the motions, not thinking much about how I feel.

    1   2   3   4   5

UFO 29

1. When I don't have a chance to exercise, I feel tremendous guilt.

    1   2   3   4   5

2. I've made exercise a priority (my workouts always come first).

    1   2   3   4   5

3. I often get anxious and irritable if I don't have a chance to work out.

    1   2   3   4   5

4. I won't take a break if I'm injured or ill (there's no excuse not to work out).

    1   2   3   4   5

5. I rarely look forward to working out, but it's something I *have* to do.

    1   2   3   4   5

6. No matter how tired or lazy I feel, I'll push myself to an extreme.

    1   2   3   4   5

UFO 30

1. I often use very heavy weights (which keeps me from using strict form).

    1   2   3   4   5

2. I care much more about how I look than I do about how I feel.

    1   2   3   4   5

3. On days when I don't look my best, I frequently skip the gym.

    1   2   3   4   5

4. I often defend my actions and will rarely admit that I'm wrong.

     1   2   3   4   5

5. I frequently argue with others about the right and wrong ways to work out.

     1   2   3   4   5

6. I'm always comparing the way I look to photos in magazines.

     1   2   3   4   5

UFO 31

1. When I try to recall what I've had to eat (during the day), my mind goes blank.

     1   2   3   4   5

2. I often underestimate how much food I have consumed.

     1   2   3   4   5

3. On a typical day, I "pick" a lot (and forget that it all adds up).

     1   2   3   4   5

4. On days when I think my diet is good, I find that I often gain weight.

     1   2   3   4   5

5. Often when I crave a snack and go to the cupboard (or open the fridge), I find that I've already eaten most or all of the thing I crave.

     1   2   3   4   5

6. I swear that I don't often eat very much, but others insist that I do.

     1   2   3   4   5

UFO 32

1. I'm frequently constipated and/or suffer from diarrhea.

     1   2   3   4   5

2. I have abdominal pain that is often relieved when I move my bowels.

     1   2   3   4   5

3. I move my bowels more or less often now than what is the norm (for me).

     1   2   3   4   5

4. I notice that certain foods cause bloating, stomach cramps, and/or gas, for example, fruit, caffeinated drinks, fried food, dairy products, and beer.

     1   2   3   4   5

5. I often feel sluggish and tired, particularly after eating big meals.

     1   2   3   4   5

6. Many foods don't agree with me (almost everything gives me gas!).

     1   2   3   4   5

UFO 33

1. When I gain weight, I adjust by not eating much the following day.

     1   2   3   4   5

2. I frequently run on empty (I go without food for long stretches of time).

     1   2   3   4   5

3. It's a given that I'll lose weight if I restrict how much I consume.

     1   2   3   4   5

4. A calorie is a calorie, no matter what form it takes.

     1   2   3   4   5

5. To start my day feeling energized, I eat lots of high-carb foods.

     1   2   3   4   5

6. I believe that certain foods can help my body burn more fat.

     1   2   3   4   5

UFO 34

1. My energy level soars then drops when I eat high-carb foods.

     1   2   3   4   5

2. The foods that I crave are those that affect my energy level most, i.e., cause drastic energy swings that lead to extreme fatigue.

    1   2   3   4   5

3. I often don't feel well when I eat foods that are high in carbs; for example, I get headaches, have trouble focusing, or feel faint.

    1   2   3   4   5

4. No matter how hard I exercise, I rarely lose much weight.

    1   2   3   4   5

5. I keep my energy level raised by eating high-carb foods, but I need to eat them frequently, i.e., every one or two hours.

    1   2   3   4   5

6. I often wake up feeling anxious and/or hungry during the night.

    1   2   3   4   5

UFO 35

1. My energy level is very low, and I'm often depressed or ill.

    1   2   3   4   5

2. I'm usually very sensitive to mental or physical stress and eat certain foods or use drugs to comfort myself or alleviate pain.

    1   2   3   4   5

3. It's hard for me to stay focused, even on simple, everyday tasks.

    1   2   3   4   5

4. I often crave sugar, sweets, alcohol, and foods that are made with yeast.

    1   2   3   4   5

5. I often feel anxious, hungry, tense, light-headed, and/or fatigued.

    1   2   3   4   5

6. Abrupt or frequent weather and temperature changes make me ill.

    1   2   3   4   5

UFO 36

1. Oftentimes I eat vegetables at the same time that I eat fruit.

    1   2   3   4   5

2. I often consume high-protein foods with foods high in sugar and starch.

    1   2   3   4   5

3. When mixing foods, I don't think much about what combinations are best.

    1   2   3   4   5

4. Often when I eat at restaurants, I'll try many different foods.

    1   2   3   4   5

5. The more food groups that I choose from, the more my stomach growls.

    1   2   3   4   5

6. I often take *four or more* different types of supplements at one time.

    1   2   3   4   5

UFO 37

1. Usually I take supplements based on advice that I get from friends.

    1   2   3   4   5

2. When it comes to advice about supplements, I seldom know what to believe.

    1   2   3   4   5

3. I have no idea if the products I take work well together or not.

    1   2   3   4   5

4. I often take my supplements with unbuffered vitamin C.

    1   2   3   4   5

5. I don't check to see if the supplements that I take are time released.

    1   2   3   4   5

6. In general, regarding supplements, I believe "one dose fits all."

    1   2   3   4   5

UFO 38

1. My weight serves as a barrier to intimacy (or abuse).

    1   2   3   4   5

2. I've been pressured by my parents to lose weight or get into shape.

    1   2   3   4   5

3. People have said (or still say) that I have a pretty or handsome face.

    1   2   3   4   5

4. My body is my identity (I *feel* only as good as I *look*).

    1   2   3   4   5

5. Oftentimes when I exercise, I set myself up to fail.

    1   2   3   4   5

6. I'd like to get into shape because there is someone I want to impress.

    1   2   3   4   5

UFO 39

1. I've been on a lot of diets, but none have had stable or lasting results.

    1   2   3   4   5

2. I'm often compelled to try diets that a celebrity has endorsed.

    1   2   3   4   5

3. I often lose weight quickly, but *always* gain most of it back.

    1   2   3   4   5

4. I frequently go on diets that are radical and extreme.

    1   2   3   4   5

5. I've tried using Fen-Phen, stimulant drugs, ephedra, or fasts to lose weight.

    1   2   3   4   5

6. Most of the diets I've tried have been from popular magazines.

    1   2   3   4   5

UFO 40

1. When I gain weight, I adjust by not eating much the following day.

    1   2   3   4   5

2. I live in/frequent/work at a place where I'm tempted by fattening foods.

    1   2   3   4   5

3. I frequently shop when I'm hungry and as a result buy fattening foods.

    1   2   3   4   5

4. I joined a gym that is far away from where I work or live.

    1   2   3   4   5

5. I often compare the way I look to pictures in magazines.

    1   2   3   4   5

6. I often buy sugary snack foods for my partner, spouse, or kids.

    1   2   3   4   5

UFO 41

1. I've often been told that I snore a lot and sound like I'm gasping for air.

    1   2   3   4   5

2. I rarely wake up in the morning feeling energized and refreshed.

    1   2   3   4   5

3. Most every day, I'm groggy, yawning a lot, or very fatigued.

    1   2   3   4   5

4. I usually wake many times at night but quickly go back to sleep.

    1   2   3   4   5

5. I've been told I often stop breathing, gag, make noise, or move about when asleep.

1   2   3   4   5

6. My neck is thick, I'm overweight, and/or I sleep on my back.

1   2   3   4   5

UFO 42

1. I usually can't fall asleep until well after 3 A.M.

1   2   3   4   5

2. If I didn't have to get up for work, I'd probably sleep until noon.

1   2   3   4   5

3. I'm most alert, and function best, at times when I "should" be asleep.

1   2   3   4   5

4. I've tried to change my sleep pattern, but I haven't had much success.

1   2   3   4   5

5. I often sleep late on weekends and enjoy taking naps during the day.

1   2   3   4   5

6. My energy level is often low because I don't get enough sleep.

1   2   3   4   5

UFO 43

1. I usually find it difficult to stay up past 8 P.M.

1   2   3   4   5

2. More often than not, I'm ready to get out of bed before 3 A.M.

1   2   3   4   5

3. I don't go out much in the evening (I get tired around 6 P.M.).

1   2   3   4   5

4. I often avoid social gatherings that require me to stay up late.

1   2   3   4   5

5. Because I retire so early, my family and friends get less of my time.

    1   2   3   4   5

6. For at least three months, I've been generally falling asleep before 7 P.M.

    1   2   3   4   5

UFO 44

1. Often when lying in bed, I feel an ache in my lower legs.

    1   2   3   4   5

2. Often my legs feel so restless that I have to get up and move.

    1   2   3   4   5

3. My lower legs often twitch and burn (I've been told they jerk when I sleep).

    1   2   3   4   5

4. I'm aware that one, or both, of my parents have/had this problem, too.

    1   2   3   4   5

5. This problem seems to come and go but is worse when I have caffeine.

    1   2   3   4   5

6. This problem often wakes me up or keeps me from falling asleep.

    1   2   3   4   5

UFO 45

1. I often work on the weekends and/or more than ten hours a day.

    1   2   3   4   5

2. I find it hard to set limits, delegate tasks, and let things go.

    1   2   3   4   5

3. I often fail to keep promises due to the time I spend at work.

    1   2   3   4   5

4. When I'm at home or vacationing, it's hard to forget about work.

    1   2   3   4   5

5. More often than not, I'm under stress or not in the best of health.

    1   2   3   4   5

6. I'm anxious and bored when I'm not doing work and usually can't relax.

    1   2   3   4   5

UFO 46

1. I don't know how to budget my time, plan ahead, or follow a plan.

    1   2   3   4   5

2. I'm often too busy, fatigued, overwhelmed, or distracted to work out.

    1   2   3   4   5

3. When I exercise, I feel guilty—I should do less "selfish" things with my time.

    1   2   3   4   5

4. I don't have time to exercise; too many other things always come first.

    1   2   3   4   5

5. Spending long hours at work is a higher priority than my health.

    1   2   3   4   5

6. Working out is a luxury, and it's one that I can't afford.

    1   2   3   4   5

UFO 47

1. Lately I've had poor posture and have often felt fragile or weak.

    1   2   3   4   5

2. Within the past year I've had a minor fall and fractured a bone.

    1   2   3   4   5

3. Lately I've noticed more frequent tightness and pain in my lower back.

    1   2   3   4   5

4. It's rare that I ever lift anything, and I don't exercise with weights.

    1   2   3   4   5

5. I often feel like my lower back or legs are about to give out.

    1   2   3   4   5

6. I often feel weak or achy when I spend too much time on my feet.

    1   2   3   4   5

UFO 48

1. Since taking a certain drug (or drugs), I've gradually put on weight.

    1   2   3   4   5

2. I've had some unusual symptoms since I started a certain drug.

    1   2   3   4   5

3. I've been feeling tense and anxious since I started a certain drug.

    1   2   3   4   5

4. I don't know all of the side effects of the drug (or drugs) I take.

    1   2   3   4   5

5. Twenty to ninety minutes after I take a certain drug, I often experience symptoms such as nausea, headache, and fatigue.

    1   2   3   4   5

6. Now that I'm taking a certain drug, I'm less interested in sex.

    1   2   3   4   5

UFO 49

1. I frequently get light-headed if I try to stand too fast.

    1   2   3   4   5

2. I often feel edgy or anxious when I skip or delay a meal.

    1   2   3   4   5

3. Throughout the day (more often than not), I'm irritable and fatigued.

    1   2   3   4   5

4. I'm always rushing and pushing myself, even when I'm fatigued.

    1   2   3   4   5

5. I often sense that my body is working too hard or under strain.

    1   2   3   4   5

6. I often work hard for long stretches of time (or until I run out of gas).

    1   2   3   4   5

UFO 50

1. I don't have a person or circle of friends I can trust to give me support.

    1   2   3   4   5

2. There are people who drain my energy and demand too much of my time.

    1   2   3   4   5

3. There are people I speak to often who are always putting me down.

    1   2   3   4   5

4. There are people I speak to often who are extremely self-absorbed.

    1   2   3   4   5

5. My partner or spouse is fearful that I'll change too much (or leave) and undermines my attempts to exercise and/or lose weight.

    1   2   3   4   5

6. Oftentimes people say or do things to sabotage my success.

    1   2   3   4   5

UFO 51

1. It's hard for me to trust advice or ask anyone for help.

    1   2   3   4   5

2. If I want something done correctly, I'm inclined to do it myself.

    1   2   3   4   5

3. The way I've been raised (or my ego) often keeps me from asking for help.

    1   2   3   4   5

4. I enjoy the challenge of solving difficult problems by myself.

    1   2   3   4   5

5. I'm afraid that if I ask for help, I'm not going to like what I hear.

    1   2   3   4   5

6. Because I'm somewhat of an introvert, I'd rather do things myself.

    1   2   3   4   5

UFO 52

1. I've been in abusive relationships and gained a lot of weight.

    1   2   3   4   5

2. When I lose weight, I feel vulnerable and usually gain it back.

    1   2   3   4   5

3. When somebody is attracted to me, I often feel unsafe.

    1   2   3   4   5

4. When somebody tries to get close to me, I'm much more apt to binge.

    1   2   3   4   5

5. It seems like the more I like someone, the more likely I am to gain weight.

    1   2   3   4   5

6. It seems that the more I fear someone, the more likely I am to gain weight.

    1   2   3   4   5

UFO 53

1. It's rare that I ever sleep soundly, and I often don't get enough sleep.

    1   2   3   4   5

2. If I don't drink coffee or drinks with caffeine, I seldom feel fully awake.

> 1   2   3   4   5

3. It seems like I'm always yawning and could easily take a nap.

> 1   2   3   4   5

4. At the end of a day I'm exhausted and head straight for the bed (or couch).

> 1   2   3   4   5

5. Lately at work I haven't been able to focus as well as I'd like.

> 1   2   3   4   5

6. I often forget or misplace things, like my cell phone, wallet, and keys.

> 1   2   3   4   5

UFO 54

1. In general, when something good happens, I brace for something bad.

> 1   2   3   4   5

2. People will think that I'm arrogant if I don't I downplay my success.

> 1   2   3   4   5

3. I believe that if I don't feel pain, I'm not going to see any gain.

> 1   2   3   4   5

4. Because the world is a dangerous place, I don't like to take many risks.

> 1   2   3   4   5

5. I'm often obliged to help others before I take any time for myself.

> 1   2   3   4   5

6. People will hate, reject, or criticize me if I look "too good."

> 1   2   3   4   5

UFO 55

1. I spend lots of time and work harder on parts of my body that have more fat.

> 1   2   3   4   5

2. I'm afraid that I'll bulk up if I train too hard or use heavy weights.

    1   2   3   4   5

3. I'm afraid that if I work out too much my appetite will increase.

    1   2   3   4   5

4. I train at a lower intensity in order to burn more fat.

    1   2   3   4   5

5. I use light weights and do more reps to tone and burn more fat.

    1   2   3   4   5

6. I often lift weights "explosively" to improve my performance in sports.

    1   2   3   4   5

UFO 56

1. I often judge myself harshly and obsess about how I look.

    1   2   3   4   5

2. My need to do everything perfectly often makes me put things off (for example, getting myself to the gym or changing the way I eat).

    1   2   3   4   5

3. If I can't do a perfect workout, I won't do one at all.

    1   2   3   4   5

4. When I work out, I often wear loose clothes to hide my flaws.

    1   2   3   4   5

5. I often dwell on what is wrong instead of what is right.

    1   2   3   4   5

6. People have often told me that I'm much too hard on myself.

    1   2   3   4   5

UFO 57

1. If I don't eat every four hours, I often feel dizzy and weak.

    1   2   3   4   5

2. Whenever I eat lots of foods that are high in carbs, I have energy swings.

    1   2   3   4   5

3. I often yawn continuously until I have some food.

    1   2   3   4   5

4. I often feel foggy headed and my vision is sometimes blurred.

    1   2   3   4   5

5. Sometimes I get so hungry that I'll eat anything I can find.

    1   2   3   4   5

6. Whenever I take long trips (by car), I have to stop often to eat.

    1   2   3   4   5

UFO 58

1. My shoulders appear to be rounded or my back is excessively arched.

    1   2   3   4   5

2. I participated in contact sports or was active in my youth.

    1   2   3   4   5

3. I often experience headaches, backaches, numbness, or pain in my joints.

    1   2   3   4   5

4. I've been in an auto accident or been injured playing a sport.

    1   2   3   4   5

5. I often suffer from colds, sinus pain, sore throats, earaches, or the flu.

    1   2   3   4   5

6. I often have pain that radiates from my back to muscles and joints.

    1   2   3   4   5

Determine your total score for each *individual* UFO (add the numbers you've circled for each of the sections of the test). Then list your top ten UFO scores with the highest ones listed first. For example, if you scored a 30 for UFO 5, put "5" at the top. If you scored 29 for UFO 12, then put "10" next on your list. If your scores turned out to be the same for two or more UFOs, go back and revisit your answers to the statements for those UFOs. If after reviewing your answers some of your scores remain the same, use your instincts to determine which UFO should be listed first. Once your UFO list is complete, review the key on the following pages. Next to the number for each UFO write the problem that must be addressed.

Example:

	Total Score	UFO Number	UFO Type
1.	30	5	Leaky Gut Syndrome
2.	29	12	Bulimia

	Total Score	UFO Number	UFO Type
1.	_____	_____	_____
2.	_____	_____	_____
3.	_____	_____	_____
4.	_____	_____	_____
5.	_____	_____	_____
6.	_____	_____	_____
7.	_____	_____	_____
8.	_____	_____	_____
9.	_____	_____	_____
10.	_____	_____	_____

UFO IDENTIFICATION KEY

UFO 1	Cortisol Imbalance
UFO 2	DHEA Imbalance
UFO 3	Low Testosterone
UFO 4	Estrogen Dominance (Women)
UFO 5	Leaky Gut Syndrome
UFO 6	Hypochlorhydria
UFO 7	Candidiasis (Candida Related Complex)
UFO 8	Hypothyroidism
UFO 9	Seasonal Affective Disorder (SAD)
UFO 10	Premenstrual Dysphoric Disorder (PMDD)
UFO 11	Attention Deficit Disorder (ADD)
UFO 12	Bulimia
UFO 13	Anorexia Nervosa
UFO 14	Body Dysmorphic Disorder (BDD)
UFO 15	Dysthymia (Low-Grade Depression)
UFO 16	Food Allergies
UFO 17	Food Intolerances
UFO 18	Multiple Chemical Sensitivities (MCS)
UFO 19	Seasonal Allergies
UFO 20	Electromagnetic Illness
UFO 21	Energy Blocks/Reversals
UFO 22	Weak Boundaries
UFO 23	"Cantdoenza" (Self-Defeating Beliefs)
UFO 24	Negative Associations with Exercise
UFO 25	"Victimitis"
UFO 26	Improper Exercise Technique
UFO 27	Overtraining
UFO 28	Undertraining
UFO 29	Exercise Addiction

CHAPTER TWO

ADDRESSING YOUR UFOs

The way I see it, if you want the rainbow,
you gotta deal with the rain.
　　　　　　　　DOLLY PARTON

Now that you know what your UFOs are, it's time to start shrinking your list. Please note that once "number one" is addressed, you may want to retake the test (often once one UFO disappears, others cease to exist). For example, if sleep debt is your top UFO and you're also depressed, it's possible that your mood will improve once you start getting better sleep.

Consider the following general guidelines for conquering your UFOs. Bear in mind that these guidelines do not represent all the options you have. They are only meant to give you a general sense of where to begin. And regarding all recommendations, remember to talk to your doctor first! This information is not to be used in place of your doctor's advice.

UFO 1: CORTISOL IMBALANCE

Cortisol (hydrocortisone) is a hormone produced in the brain, the level of which increases when we feel threatened or under stress. A chronic high cortisol level can cause weight gain and fatigue, as well as depression, muscle mass loss, insomnia, and thin skin. Other symptoms are feeling on edge, swollen or painful joints, hypertension, low body temperature, increased sugar cravings, and rapid pulse.

Recommendations
1. Take Phosphatidylserine or acetyl-L-carnitine. For advice about taking these supplements, see a doctor or naturopath.
2. To find out your cortisol level, take a blood or saliva test. Some experts feel that it's better to test saliva rather than blood, as its measure of "active" cortisol in your body is more precise.

3. To lower your cortisol level and reduce your level of stress, experts suggest at least three aerobic workouts every week.

4. Ask your doctor if taking GABA is worth a try. GABA, an amino acid–like antianxiety aid, is often prescribed to elevate mood and reduce the effects of stress. *Note:* If you're taking an antidepressant, *don't* take GABA (before taking *any* supplement, consult a medical doctor or naturopath).

5. Don't overtrain (it can cause your cortisol level to increase). A saliva test can help to reveal if your body is overtrained. If three hours after you train you find that your cortisol level is raised, you'll need to shorten your workout, train less often, or get more rest.

6. Drink water! (Dehydration can raise cortisol levels, too.)

7. Reduce your consumption of sugar, yeast, and highly processed foods. Since cortisol raises blood sugar, which can increase the growth of yeast, there is a good chance that candidiasis (yeast overgrowth) will occur.

8. To lower your cortisol level, limit your intake of caffeine.

Books

Safe Uses of Cortisol by William McK Jefferies, M.D. Charles C. Thomas Pub. Ltd., 1996.

Web Links

http://stress.about.com/library/weekly/aa012901a.htm
http://my.webmd.com/content/article/1728.69924
www.nlm.nih.gov/medlineplus/ency/article/003693.htm

UFO 2: DHEA IMBALANCE

DHEA is a hormone that decreases as we age, often most noticeably around the age of thirty-five. (Research has shown that between the ages of twenty and sixty-five DHEA levels typically drop as much as 80 percent!)

DHEA is often believed to have antiaging effects. It also helps prevent cancer, hypertension, and tumor growth, as well as thyroid dysfunction, anxiety, bone loss, and fatigue. Additionally, this hormone can aid in increasing muscle mass and prevent radiation damage from electrical fields or the sun.

Recommendations

1. Stop (or decrease significantly) tobacco and alcohol use. Habitual use will lower your overall level of DHEA.

2. If you are taking birth control pills, change the type or dose. Taking the wrong medication or dose can lower your DHEA.

3. Ask your doctor if you should test your level of DHEA.

4. Avoid steroids unless prescribed for specific health concerns. Steroid use can slow or halt the production of DHEA.

5. Ask your medical doctor if you should take DHEA. Typically, DHEA is prescribed for four to six weeks at a time, as most doctors feel that taking it longer than this can pose a risk (adrenal dysfunction, anxiety, liver toxicity, and fatigue).

Books

All About DHEA: Frequently Asked Questions by Ray Sahelian and Jack Challem. Avery Penguin Putnam, 1999.

The DHEA Breakthrough by Stephen A. Cherniske. Ballantine Books, 1998.

Web Links

www.ceri.com/dhea.htm
www.biopsychiatry.com/dhea.htm

UFO 3: LOW TESTOSTERONE

If lately you've struggled to gain muscle mass, lose weight, or increase your strength, a hormone imbalance, or low testosterone level, may be the cause. Here are some symptoms of low testosterone (do any apply?):

- Low levels of HDL (good cholesterol) and high levels of LDL (bad cholesterol)
- Elevated insulin levels (causing your body to store more fat)
- High blood pressure that doesn't respond very well to reductions in stress
- Increased abdominal fat (increasing the risk of poor cardiac health)
- Consistent bouts of fatigue and the need for increased amounts of sleep
- Depression, dulled senses, lethargy, low motivation, and lack of pep
- Premature aging, lines in the face, loose skin, and graying hair

- Diminished sexual performance and reduced interest in sex
- Brittle bones, muscle soreness, increased healing time, and nagging pains
- Decreased muscle mass or endurance, and a gradual gain in weight

Even if your total testosterone level is in the right range, your level of *free* testosterone might still be abnormally low. The "free" form of testosterone is what binds to receptors in cells, unless they're suppressed by sex hormone–binding globulin (SHBG). Excess estrogen often can boost the production of SHBG, as can the aging process and the use of some birth control pills.

Recommendations

1. Ask your physician if you should take a "free" testosterone test. This is the best indicator of whether you need a replacement drug. It's important to ask about testing other hormone levels, too, such as thyroid, estrogen, cortisol, adrenal function, and DHEA.
2. You may have a zinc deficiency if your testosterone level is low. See a homeopath or holistic nutritionist for advice.

Books

The Testosterone Syndrome: The Critical Factor for Energy, Health, and Sexuality—Reversing the Male Menopause by Eugene Shippen, M.D., and William Fryer. M. Evans and Co., 1998.

The Testosterone Revolution: Rediscover Your Energy and Overcome the Symptoms of Male Menopause by Malcolm Carruthers. Thorsons, 2001.

The Testosterone Solution: Increase Your Energy and Vigor with Male Hormone Therapy by Aubrey M. Hill. Prima Publishing, 1998.

Web Links

www.urologychannel.com/testosteronedeficiency/index.shtml
www.duj.com/article/hellstrom2/hellstrom2.html
www.e-testosterone.net

UFO 4: ESTROGEN DOMINANCE (WOMEN)

If a blood or saliva test reveals that your estrogen level is high, estrogen dominance may be one of your primary UFOs. Estrogen dominance causes anxiety, mood swings, and fatigue. Too much estrogen also can cause aldosterone levels to rise, which leads to fluid retention, abdominal swelling, and swollen breasts.

Many experts contend that when estrogen levels are very high, a low pro-gesterone level is likely to be the primary cause. Other possible causes are the consumption of sugar-rich foods, a vitamin B_6 deficiency, a low-fiber diet, and liver disease.

Recommendations

1. Ask your physician if you should take black cohosh or St. John's wort. These herbs are often prescribed for women with chronic PMS. They have also been found to be helpful to women with symptoms of menopause.
2. Ask your physician if taking estriol is worth a try. According to some physicians, estriol is the treatment of choice (it generally has fewer side effects and contributes to vaginal health).
3. Find out about natural progesterone, evening primrose oil, and B_6. According to many doctors, progesterone creams work especially well.
4. Selective serotonin reuptake inhibitors (SSRIs) can help. They include drugs such as Lexapro, Prozac, Paxil, and Zoloft.
5. Take magnesium, calcium, L-taurine, or lecithin. Ask a naturopath or medical doctor for advice.

Books

Women's Bodies, Women's Wisdom by Christiane Northrup, M.D. Bantam Doubleday Dell, 1998.

The Estrogen Alternative: Natural Hormone Therapy with Botanical Progesterone by Raquel Martin and Judi Gerstung. Inner Traditions Intl. Ltd., 2000.

A Woman's Guide to Natural Hormones by Christine Conrad. Perigee, 2000.

Web Links

www.4woman.gov/faq/pms.htm
www.emedicine.com/ped/topic1890.htm
www.consciouschoice.com/holisticmd/hmd1209.html

UFO 5: LEAKY GUT SYNDROME

When food "leaks" through the intestinal wall and toxins enter the blood, according to many experts, it's the result of a "leaky gut." Toxicity symptoms and nutrient malabsorption can result, which can cause a whole rash of problems, ranging from marked weight gain to fatigue.

The causes of leaky gut syndrome can be fasting or alcohol use, an autoimmune disorder, or sensitivity to certain drugs (Motrin, Advil, Naprosyn, and anticancer drugs). Pancreatic enzyme deficiencies can create this problem, too, as can a food intolerance or the consumption of toxic foods.

Recommendations

1. Ask your doctor about L-glutamine and DGL. L-glutamine is used to fortify the intestinal walls. To protect your stomach lining, experts recommend DGL (deglycyrrhizinated licorice root).
2. Ask your doctor about an intestinal permeability test. By assessing the ratio of two different sugars (lactolose and mannitol), it's possible to determine the permeability of your gut.
3. Take a stool test to evaluate your gastrointestinal health. A stool test will assess how well you absorb and break down food. It will also measure bacteria and yeast levels in your gut.
4. Create a healthy balance of bacteria in your gut. To increase the ratio of good to bad bacteria in your gut, an acidophilus supplement such as PB-8 may help.
5. Address your food sensitivities to curb gastrointestinal stress.

Books

Your Wakeup Call to Health: Part 1, The Leaky Gut Syndrome by Dr. Peggy J. Locke. Wellness Publishing, 2001.

Leaky Gut Syndrome by Elizabeth Lipski. McGraw-Hill/NTC, 1998.

Web Links

http://osiris.sunderland.ac.uk/autism/gut.htm
www.nutri-notes.com/marapr98_simple.htm
http://acudoc.com/leaky.html

UFO 6: HYPOCHLORHYDRIA

Hypochlorhydria is the underproduction of HCl (hydrochloric acid). When the stomach fails to produce an adequate level of HCl, the breakdown of protein is hindered, which can eventually cause poor health. An enzyme called pepsin also helps your stomach break down food, but not if low levels of HCl prevent it from doing its job. This problem affects more than half of people over fifty years old.

Most people with low HCl are treated as if they're producing too much, largely because the symptoms of both conditions are nearly the same (bloating, belching, heartburn, stomach pain, and excessive gas).

Recommendations

1. Ask your doctor if betaine HCl is worth a try. If you have no burning sensation and your symptoms begin to subside, your doctor may view it as proof that you're not producing enough HCl.
2. Find out if there's any undigested protein in your stools. Have a stool analysis (ask your doctor for details). Undigested protein suggests a low level of HCl.
3. Take the Heidelburg test to measure your level of HCl. This test measures how well your stomach produces HCl. It requires you to swallow a pill that transmits data to a machine (the pill contains a microchip that measures your stomach's pH). The data is used to evaluate your need for digestive aids.
4. Consider taking digestive enzyme supplements with your meals. Digestive enzymes often contain pepsin and bromelain, as well as ox bile, pancreatin, and betaine HCl (other common ingredients are amylase, papain, and protease).
5. Take glutamic acid hydrochloride with your meals. The powdered form is often preferred, as pills take more time to digest.
6. Don't take any antacids—they will just make your problem worse.

Books

Why Stomach Acid Is Good for You by Jonathan V. Wright and Lane Lenard. M. Evans and Company, Inc., 2001.

Web Links

www.medical-library.net/sites/framer.html?/sites/_hypochlorhydria.html

UFO 7: CANDIDIASIS (CANDIDA RELATED COMPLEX)

Candidiasis, or candida related complex (CRC), is a chronic, systemic infection caused by an overproduction of yeast. A diet high in sugar and yeast is typically at the root, but antibiotics and birth control pills can cause this problem as well.

When the right combination of factors lead to overproduction of yeast, it can cause an allergic reaction that sends toxins into your blood. The release of histamines is caused by yeast overgrowth as well, causing symptoms such as headaches, light-headed spells, sore throat, and fatigue.

By suppressing your immune system, triggering cravings, and causing fatigue, CRC can prevent you from losing weight and getting fit.

Recommendations

1. Ask your doctor if he or she thinks you might have CRC. Make a list of your symptoms and be sure to discuss each one. Your doctor may want to examine your stools for excessive amounts of yeast and possibly test your blood as well for signs of CRC.
2. Try a little experiment—consider rotating your foods. For example, if on a Monday you eat yeast-free bread and fish, try to wait until Friday to consume those foods again. Within the CRC guidelines (see page 199), vary your diet as much as you can.

Books

The Yeast Connection: A Medical Breakthrough by William G. Crook. Vintage Books, 1986.

The Allergy Self-Help Cookbook: Over 325 Natural Foods Recipes, Free of Wheat, Milk, Eggs, Corn, Yeast, Sugar and Other Common Food Allergens by Marjorie Hunt Jones. Rodale Press, 2001.

Special Diet Solutions: Healthy Cooking Without Wheat, Gluten, Dairy, Eggs, Yeast or Refined Sugar by Carol Lee Fenster, Ph.D. Savory Palate, 1997.

Check out the following website for a list of other books: http://depressionbookstore.com/nutrition_depression/candida

Web Links

www.infosky.net/~alexmi/candida.htm
www.colonichealth.com/candid.htm
www.intelegen.com/nutrients/candida_yeast_protection_program1.htm

UFO 8: HYPOTHYROIDISM

Hypothyroidism can be caused by a number of things, from an underactive thyroid to inadequate TSH (thyroid-stimulating hormone). A slow metabolism is the most frequently cited result, but symptoms can also include a low energy level and chronic fatigue. People who have this problem also complain of being cold and tend to suffer from illnesses more frequently than the norm.

Recommendations

1. Hypothyroidism can be confirmed with various tests. Talk to your doctor about taking tests that measure T3 and T4. T3 and T4 are hormones that are produced by the thyroid gland (T3, or triiodthyronine, is four times as strong as T4, but the thyroid produces four times as much thyroxine, i.e., T4). A radioimmunoassay is the best-known thyroid test, but there are other tests as well that your doctor may suggest. These tests include iodine uptake scans, biopsies, and ultrasound, as well as those that measure TBG and TRH (thyroid-binding globulin and TSH–releasing hormone).

2. Ask your doctor if you should be taking thyroid hormone drugs. Levothyroxine, also known as Synthroid, may be prescribed. Cytomel (triiodothyronine) may be recommended, too. A full response to this therapy can take up to one or two months, but a slight reduction in symptoms should be noted within a week.

3. Find out if you are deficient in iodine or zinc. A selenium deficiency can cause thyroid problems, too. Consider taking a blood test to determine where you stand.

Books

Thyroid Power: Ten Steps to Total Health by Richard Shames, M.D., Karilee Halo, R.N., and Nathan Becker. Harper Resource, 2001.

Living Well with Hypothyroidism: What Your Doctor Doesn't Tell You . . . That You Need to Know by Mary J. Shomon. Wholecare, 2000.

The Thyroid Solution: A Mind-Body Program for Beating Depression and Regaining Your Emotional and Physical Health by Ridha Arem, M.D. Ballantine Books, 2000.

Web Links

www.endocrineweb.com/hypo1.html
http://my.webmd.com/content/article/1680.51476

UFO 9: SEASONAL AFFECTIVE DISORDER (SAD)

If you get more depressed in the fall and winter months, you may have SAD (seasonal affective disorder). Symptoms include depression, increased appetite, and excessive sleep, as well as weight gain, increased carbohydrate cravings, and daytime fatigue. This problem is easily treated with the use of full-spectrum lights.

Recommendations

1. Find out if you really have SAD by taking a simple test. The Seasonal Pattern Assessment Questionnaire (SPAQ) is the test that most practitioners use to diagnose SAD. To assess the extent to which people react negatively to seasonal change, the Hamilton Rating Scale for SAD is also used. This test is often used to confirm the results of the SPAQ. For additional information, look at the following link: www.normanrosenthal.com/winter_blues_2.html.

2. Find out if an antidepressant could provide the help you need. Selective serotonin reuptake inhibitors, also called SSRIs, have proved to be very effective for those who suffer from SAD. SSRIs include Lexapro, Prozac, Paxil, and Zoloft.

3. Try out a dawn simulator, bright-light visor, or light box. Parameters for light therapy are wavelength and intensity (lux), as well as the time of day and amount of time that the light is used. The intensity is generally 2,500 to 10,000 lux, and the length of time to use the light is about one hour a day (for some people, thirty minutes will provide a good response). Ultraviolet wavelengths should be filtered out of the light, and full strength, white fluorescent bulbs should be the only source. If you can't afford a light box, you can use full-spectrum bulbs. When placed in overhead lights or lamps in your bedroom, office, or home, full-spectrum bulbs can have benefits that compare to using a box. Some response to light therapy should be seen within two to four days, but a noticeable improvement should be observed within a week. Common side effects are nausea, headache, and eyestrain, but these problems are usually quickly resolved by viewing the light for less time.

4. Experiment with the position in which you place your bright-light source. While some people have a better response when the source is straight ahead, others benefit more when it is raised or off to the side. Also, the light should generally be about 3 feet from your eyes.

Books

Winter Blues: Seasons of the Mind: Why You Get the Winter Blues & What You Can Do About It by Norman E. Rosenthal, M.D. Guilford Press, 1993.

Fight the Winter Blues—Don't Be Sad: Your Guide to Conquering Seasonal Affective Disorder by Celeste A. Peters. Script Publishing, 1994.

Web Links

www.mentalhealth.com/book/p40-sad.html
www.phothera.com/ptfaq.html

For details about purchasing a bright light, check out the following links:

www.lighttherapyproducts.com
www.lifestyler.com/superlamp
www.apollolight.com
www.phothera.com/index.html
www.soleilsunalarm.com
www.biobrite.com
www.healthlight.net

UFO 10: PREMENSTRUAL DYSPHORIC DISORDER (PMDD)

Premenstrual dysphoric disorder is an extreme form of PMS. If you happen to have PMDD but don't think that it's a big deal, there's a pretty good chance that your coworkers, family, and friends have a contrary view.

Recurrent problems with PMS can keep you from getting in shape. It's hard enough to eat healthy and get to the gym when you're feeling good, so it follows that mood and energy swings, when severe, could affect your resolve. Symptoms of PMDD include anxiety and tender breasts, as well as sleep disturbances, irritability, and fatigue.

Recommendations

1. Selective serotonin reuptake inhibitors (SSRIs) can help. They include drugs such as Lexapro, Prozac, Paxil, and Zoloft. Consult your physician for more information about how these drugs can help.
2. An antiestrogenic hormone drug may be your "cure." Ask your physician if taking a drug is appropriate in your case.
3. Do more aerobic exercise to keep symptoms under control.
4. Ask your physician if there are alternative treatments you can try, such as primrose oil, B_6, and natural progesterone. Calcium and

magnesium may alleviate symptoms, too, but before you take any supplements seeing your doctor is strongly advised.

Books

Women's Bodies, Women's Wisdom: Creating Physical and Emotional Health and Healing by Christiane Northrup, M.D. Bantam Books, 1990.

Dr. Susan Lark's Premenstrual Syndrome Self-Help Book: A Woman's Guide to Feeling Good All Month by Susan Lark, M.D. Celestial Arts, 1989.

Screaming to Be Heard: Hormonal Connections Women Suspect, and Doctors Still Ignore by Elizabeth Lee Vliet, M.D. M. Evans and Company, Inc. 2001.

Web Links

www.usdoctor.com/pms.htm
www.womanshealthonline.net/article1037.html
www.nlm.nih.gov/medlineplus/menstruationandpremenstrualsyndrome.html

To see if you have PMDD, check the following link:

www.womens-health.org/pmdd.html

UFO 11: ATTENTION DEFICIT DISORDER (ADD)

If you're impulsive, often distracted, unfocused, and easily bored, attention deficit disorder (ADD) may be the cause. Other symptoms are talking too much, forgetting important things, fidgeting, feeling restless, and failing to finish important tasks.

Four to 6 percent of adults are thought to have ADD. If you have ADD and you find it hard to diet or get to the gym, it will probably *always* be hard for you if this problem is not addressed.

It's important to note that you don't have to be hyperactive to have ADD. Although most ADD sufferers are unfocused much of the time, they also can be hyperfocused, i.e., they can be at either extreme.

Recommendations

1. If your ADD is severe, consider getting medical help. Your doctor may prescribe Wellbutrin (an antidepressant drug), which can stabilize neurotransmitters related to ADD. Paradoxically, stimulant drugs (such as Ritalin) can be effective, too.

2. Learn how to be more focused by getting help from an ADD coach. See the Web Links for referrals (coaching is often done over the phone).

3. Use meditation or counseling to get symptoms under control. Behavior and cognitive therapy is a good way to address ADD.

Books

Healing ADD: The Breakthrough Program That Allows You to See and Heal the Six Types of ADD by Daniel Amen, M.D. Putnam Pub Group, 2001.

Driven to Distraction by Edward M. Hallowell, M.D., and John J. Ratey, M.D. Pantheon, 1994.

Out of the Fog: Treatment Options and Coping Strategies for Adult ADD by Kevin R. Murphy and Suzanne LeVert. Hyperion, 1995.

Web Links

www.add.org
www.oneaddplace.com
www.attentiondeficitdisorder.ws

Interactive tests for adult ADD:

www.amenclinic.com/ac/addtests/adult.asp
www.psychologynet.org/symadd.html

For coaching referrals:

www.comprehensivecoachingu.com/referral/searchdetail.lasso

UFO 12: BULIMIA

The symptoms of bulimia are strict dieting, swollen glands, preoccupation with body weight, and purging after a binge. Bulimics are often obsessed with gaining control of their weight and food and driven to make themselves thin without regard for their physical health.

Bulimics may use ephedra or diuretics to lose weight and may have irregular periods, dental problems, and frequent colds. Certain activities can be a trigger for this disease as well, including gymnastics, modeling, long-distance running, and working in gyms.

Medical complications include:

- Erosion of tooth enamel caused by the acids in bile during a purge
- Electrolyte imbalance, dehydration, and swollen glands
- Frequent irregular heartbeat, palpitations, or panic attacks

Recommendations

1. Cognitive and behavioral psychotherapy is advised.
2. Consider medical treatment, i.e., an antidepressant drug. Selective serotonin reuptake inhibitors (SSRIs) work well and are often the treatment of choice when bulimia symptoms are severe. Examples are Prozac (fluoxetine) and Lexapro (escitalopram).
3. Group therapy can be effective, especially for young adults.
4. An eating disorders program may provide the help you need. Look into treatment centers that provide long-term support.

Books

Breaking Free from Compulsive Eating by Geneen Roth. Signet, 1984.

Feeding the Hungry Heart: The Experience of Compulsive Eating by Geneen Roth. Signet, 1982.

Web Links

www.nami.org/helpline/bulimia.html
www.1-800-therapist.com
www.anad.org

UFO 13: ANOREXIA NERVOSA

Anorexia nervosa is a fear of becoming fat, characterized by distortions of one's size and physical flaws. Compulsive exercise is a common result of this disease, as well as self-starvation, amenorrhea (absence of menstruation), and failing health. Denial of one's situation is also a hallmark of this disease, in addition to "secret behaviors" such as purging after a meal. Untreated, this problem is serious and can even lead to death, as hormonal problems and heartbeat abnormalities can result (low serum potassium levels affect the rhythm and health of the heart).

If others have voiced concern about your lifestyle, health, and weight, consider the following symptoms (if they apply, seek professional help):

- A persistent, staunch refusal to maintain a normal weight
- A distorted view of one's size and shape (perceiving oneself as fat)
- The absence of three consecutive menstrual cycles (amenorrhea)
- A weight loss of more than 15 percent of one's normal, healthy weight

Recommendations

1. Review the treatment options advised for bulimia (UFO 12).
2. Find a good support group (one where you won't feel pressured or judged). By hearing what others have to say, you'll feel less confused and alone.

Books

Thin Disguise: Understanding and Overcoming Anorexia and Bulimia by Pam Vredevelt, Deborah Newman, Harry Beverly, and Frank Minirth. Nelson, 1992.

Hunger Pains—From Fad Diets to Eating Disorders: What Every Woman Needs to Know About Food, Dieting, and Self-Concept by Mary Pipher. Adams Publishing, 1995.

Web Links

www.nami.org/helpline/anorexia.htm
www.anad.org
www.findinfo.com/anorexia.htm
www.edreferral.com
www.1-800-therapist.com

Treatment Centers

The Renfrew Center: www.renfrew.org

Johns Hopkins Eating Disorders Center: www.med.jhu.edu/jhhpsychiatry/ed1.htm

The Meadows: www.themeadows.org

UFO 14: BODY DYSMORPHIC DISORDER (BDD)

If you focus a lot on your physical flaws, even though others think you look fine, you may have a problem called body dysmorphic disorder (BDD). People with BDD are often obsessed about how they look; for example, they fear that their nose is too big or their chest (or breasts) too small.

People with this disorder often try to hide their "flaws," for example, by using makeup, tensing their muscles, or wearing loose clothes. Additionally, they tend to look in the mirror more than the norm and scrutinize photos in magazines to obsess about how they compare.

Recommendations

1. Selective serotonin reuptake inhibitors (SSRIs) can help. They include drugs such as Prozac, Lexapro, Paxil, and Zoloft. Consult your physician for more information about how these drugs are used.
2. Consider seeing a therapist to get symptoms under control. Behavior and cognitive therapy is a good way to address BDD.

Books

The Adonis Complex: The Secret Crisis of Male Body Obsession by Harrison G. Pope, Jr., M.D., Katharine A. Phillips, M.D., and Roberto Olivardia, Ph.D. Touchstone Books, 2002.

The Broken Mirror: Understanding and Treating Body Dysmorphic Disorder by Katharine A. Phillips, M.D. Oxford University Press, 1998.

Web Links

www.butler.org/bdd
www.nami.org/youth/dysmorphic.html
www.emedicine.com/med/topic3124.htm

Online support group:

www.e-groups.com/group/bodydysmorphic

UFO 15: DYSTHYMIA (LOW-GRADE DEPRESSION)

Depression can be the result of drug interactions or lack of sleep. It can also be the result of more "obvious" things such as problems at work, addictions, relationship challenges, lifestyle issues, and chronic stress.

Remember, if you're depressed, you'll be more apt to skip the gym, your energy level will suffer, and you'll be prone to overeat. And although working out can boost your mood—as long as you're not too depressed—the paradox is that if you're depressed, you're not going to want to work out (finding the motivation to train is hard enough when you feel good!).

1. If you're clearly depressed (and it's been a while), get some medical help. If you're predisposed to depression and have an imbalance affecting your brain, it's unlikely that simply "talking it out" will do very much to help. This is akin to discussing the cause of a rapidly sinking ship, which is okay to do if the ship isn't actually sinking while you're aboard! Once you know that a hole is there and the water is filling your boat, the hole must be patched before you discuss any thoughts about how it occurred. Antidepressants are often the best (and most sensible) way to go, provided the one that you take is the dosage and type that is best for you.
2. Talk to your doctor about SAM-e, St. John's wort, and 5-HTP.
3. Take omega-3 supplements (fish or flax oil) every day.
4. Find out if a food allergy (or the way you've been eating) has made you depressed.
5. Address your suppressed emotions, in particular, guilt and rage. Conventional psychotherapy is a pretty good place to start, but energy block acutherapy (EBA) can also help.
6. Find out what other UFOs are making you feel depressed: for example, sleep debt, allergens, drug interactions, or chronic fatigue.

Books

Undoing Depression: What Therapy Doesn't Teach You and Medication Can't Give You by Richard O'Connor. Berkley Publishing Group, 1999.

Feeling Good: The New Mood Therapy by David Burns, M.D. Wholecare, 1999.

You Mean, I Don't Have to Feel This Way? New Help for Depression, Anxiety, and Addiction by Colette Dowling. Scribner, 1991.

Nutrition and Mental Illness: An Orthomolecular Approach to Balancing Body Chemistry by Carl Curt Pfeiffer. Inner Traditions Intl. Ltd., 1988.

Web Links

To see if you are depressed:

www.depression-screening.org

For general advice and support:

www.healingwell.com/depression

www.faqs.org/faqs/alt-support-depression/faq
www.psycom.net/depression.central.html

To practice energy treatments for depression and chronic stress:

www.emofree.com

UFO 16: FOOD ALLERGIES

When we have an allergic reaction to a food that we consume, it's due to immune responses caused by allergens in that food. Food allergens are proteins that the body fails to break down, which can irritate parts of the body, triggering various types of distress. Examples are diarrhea, abdominal cramps, and an "itchy" mouth. Allergy-causing foods include legumes, shellfish, and eggs, as well as peanuts, most tree nuts, wheat products, and MSG. And since many foods contain additives, such as chemicals, hormones, and dyes, it's important to look at labels (and eat organic whenever you can).

Recommendations

1. Consider taking the ALCAT test to assess your responses to foods. For more information on how to take this test and what it entails, see the Web Links section and Rivera and Deutsch's book.
2. Take Coca's pulse test for food allergies:

   - Take your pulse before you consume the food that you wish to test.
   - Consume the food you wish to test (do not eat anything else).
   - Maintain a relaxed position in a place where you don't feel stressed.
   - Wait at least twenty minutes and then take your pulse again. If your pulse has increased by ten or more beats, an allergy may be the cause.

Books

Food Allergies and Food Intolerance: The Complete Guide to Their Identification and Treatment by Jonathan Brostoff and Linda Gamlin. Inner Traditions Intl. Ltd., 2000.

The Food Allergy Book: The Foods That Cause You Pain and Discomfort and How to Take Them Out of Your Diet by William F. Walsh and Felicia Busch. ACA Publications, Inc., 1995.

The Rotation Diet Cookbook: A 4-Day Plan for Relieving Allergies by Jill Carter and Alison Edwards. Element, 1997.

Your Hidden Food Allergies Are Making You Fat: The ALCAT Food Sensitivities Weight Loss Breakthrough by Rudy Rivera and Roger D. Deutsch. Prima Publishing, 1998.

Web Links

www.nidlink.com/~mastent
www.food-allergy.org
www.niaid.nih.gov/factsheets/food.htm

For information on the ALCAT test:

www.alcat.com
www.healthchoice.net/lab/alcat.html

UFO 17: FOOD INTOLERANCES

A food intolerance often results in lethargy and fatigue. Headaches and gastrointestinal ills are also a common result, as are flushing, bloating, increased perspiration, and rapid pulse. These symptoms can sap your energy, cause weight gain, and limit your strength.

More often than not, the foods that we crave are the ones we tolerate least. When it comes to prime offenders, wheat and yeast products head the list, followed by dairy foods, including yogurt, milk, and eggs.

Recommendations

1. Consider the following supplements (but check with your doctor first):

   - *MSM* has been found to help keep cravings under control. See the Web Links section for more information about MSM (methyl sulfonyl methane, often used for pain relief).
   - *Fibercon*, or any good fiber supplement, taken with food.

2. If you are lactose intolerant, only buy foods that are lactose free.
3. Avoid or consume very sparingly any foods you're intolerant of.

Books

Was It Something You Ate? Food Intolerance—What Causes It and How to Avoid It by John Emsley and Peter Fell. Oxford University Press, Inc., 1999.

Food Allergies and Food Intolerance: The Complete Guide to Their Identification and Treatment by Jonathan Brostoff and Linda Gamlin. Inner Traditions Intl. Ltd., 2000.

Web Links

www.niaid.nih.gov/factsheets/food.htm
http://users.bigpond.net.au/allergydietitian/fa_fl_food_intolerance.html
www.skyisland.com/onlineresources

For information about MSM:

www.arthritis-msm-supplements.com
www.bulkmsm.com/default.html
www.worldimage.com/products/info/msm/msmfacts.html

UFO 18: MULTIPLE CHEMICAL SENSITIVITIES (MCS)

Common MCS symptoms are feeling light-headed and fatigued, as well as achy, irritable, disoriented, and faint. Insomnia, memory problems, and migraine headaches are common as well, as are rashes, nausea, constipation, and ringing ears.

MCS appears to affect young women most of all. If you think that you have this problem, you'll need help to determine the cause.

Recommendations

1. Use unscented lotions, creams, hair products, soaps, and sprays.
2. Avoid using any home or office products with chemical scents. This includes air freshener, furniture polish, and window spray.
3. Take steps to improve the air quality in your office, car, and home. Use air-conditioning filters and replace them every two months. Purchase an air purifier (and make sure that you keep it clean). Make sure that your windows are closed when sitting in traffic (and close your vents!).

Books

My House Is Killing Me! The Home Guide for Families with Allergies and Asthma by Jeffrey C. May and Jonathan M. Samet. Johns Hopkins University Press, 2001.

Chemical Sensitivity: Environmental Diseases and Pollutants—How They Hurt Us and How to Deal with Them by Sherry Rogers. McGraw-Hill/NTC, 2001.

Multiple Chemical Sensitivity: A Survival Guide by Pamela Reed Gibson, Ph.D. New Harbinger, 2000.

Web Links

www.aaem.com
www.naet.com
www.mcsurvivors.com
www.sw.org/poison/multchem.htm

UFO 19: SEASONAL ALLERGIES

Thirty-five million Americans suffer from allergies every year. Avoiding what you're allergic to is often suggested first, followed by medication, allergy tests, and allergy shots.

Recommendations

1. Ask your doctor if taking corticosteroids is advised. They help to reduce inflammation when applied to your nose or eyes.
2. Find out if you should have allergy tests and if you need allergy shots.
3. Ask your doctor if antihistamines are worth a try.
4. Keep all doors and windows shut in your office, car, and home.
5. Wash your hair and hands often when you spend any time outdoors.

Books

The Allergy Sourcebook: Everything You Need to Know by Merla Zellerbach and Vincent A. Marinkovich. McGraw-Hill/NTC, 2000.

Allergy-Free Naturally: 1,000 Non-Drug Solutions for More Than 50 Allergy-Related Problems by Rick Ansorge and Eric Metcalf. Rodale Press, 2001.

Indoor Air Quality Handbook by John D. Spengler, John F. McCarthy, and Jonathan M. Samet (Eds.). McGraw-Hill Professional Publishing, 2000.

UFO 20: ELECTROMAGNETIC ILLNESS

If you frequently use a computer, microwave oven, or cellular phone, you're affected by radiation from electromagnetic fields. Transformers, high-tension wires, and electrical plants can cause problems as well, which is why we all need to take steps to avoid radiation as much as we can.

Electromagnetic illness can cause facial flushing and problems with sleep, in addition to nausea, dizziness, muscle spasms, and marked fatigue. Add to the list brain fog, headaches, skin rashes, earaches, and dry eyes, and it's easy to see how a problem like this can be a UFO.

Recommendations

1. Avoid radiation sources, such as computers and cellular phones. Limit your use of these items or protect yourself (see below).
2. Make sure your computer monitor has an antistatic screen. The screen should be grounded (attached to a metal object by a wire).
3. Replace your computer monitor—purchase one with an LCD. LCDs (liquid crystal displays) are safer than CRTs (cathode-ray tubes).
4. Purchase a radiation protection case for your cellular phone (see Web Links).
5. Inspect the areas near your bed and desk for unshielded wires. Also check to see if electrical outlets are near your bed. If this is the case, try moving your bed to a different place in your room.
6. Unplug any lamps or electrical items prior to going to sleep, or use an extension cord to plug them in somewhere else in the room.
7. To determine where there are high radiation levels in your home, use an electromagnetic detection device to expose the source. The WiN-RADiO ERD-1500 is an example of such a device (see Web Links).

Books

Cross Currents: The Perils of Electropollution/The Promise of Electromedicine by Robert O. Becker. Jeremy Tarcher, 1990.

Health Hazards of Electromagnetic Radiation: A Startling Look at the Effects of Electropollution on Your Health by Bruce Fife. Piccadilly Books, 1998.

Biological Effects of Electric and Magnetic Fields: Sources and Mechanisms by David O. Carpenter and Sinerik Ayrapetyan (Eds.). Academic Press, 1994.

Your UFOs

Web Links

www.idcnet.com/~jschultz/es.htm
www.niehs.nih.gov/emfrapid/home.htm
www.emrnetwork.org
www.protect-o-cell.com
www.xternet.de/bioelektrik/protector/phone-case.htm
www.lessemf.com/cellphon.html
www.winradio.com/home/erd.htm

UFO 21: ENERGY BLOCKS/REVERSALS

See Chapter Seven to learn about how to overcome energy blocks.

Books

Instant Emotional Healing by George J. Pratt and Peter T. Lambrou. Broadway Books, 2000.

Tapping the Healer Within: Using Thought Field Therapy to Instantly Conquer Your Fears, Anxieties, and Emotional Distress by Roger Callahan, Ph.D., Richard Trubo, and Earl Mindell. Contemporary Books, 2001.

Energy Diagnostic and Treatment Methods by Fred Gallo. W. W. Norton & Co., 2000.

Web Links

www.tftrx.com (Official site of Roger Callahan, Ph.D., the creator of thought field therapy. E-mail Dr. Callahan at Roger@tftrx.com.)
www.psychinnovations.com
www.emofree.com (emotional freedom techniques)
www.energypsych.com

UFO 22: WEAK BOUNDARIES

If you tend to let people get to you or have a hard time saying no, developing stronger boundaries may be a key to improving your health. People who have weak boundaries often don't have time for themselves, mainly because they feel pressured to give their attention to others first. For example, they may miss a workout to assist a needy friend or allow someone to be critical of their style of dress or weight.

Recommendations

1. Go to an Al-Anon meeting for some encouragement and support.
2. Find a therapist you can trust or hire a professional coach.
3. Let all your boundary bashers know that the jig is officially up! Learn where to draw the line and be committed to keeping it firm. An example of what you might say is, "So I can take better care of myself, I'm not going to be as available as I have been in the past." Or, "What you said feels critical, so it's important to me that you stop."

Books

Stand Up for Your Life: Develop the Courage, Confidence, and Character to Fulfill Your Greatest Potential by Cheryl Richardson. Free Press, 2002.

Boundaries by Dr. Henry Cloud and Dr. John Townsend. Zondervan Publishing House, 1992.

Facing Codependence: What It Is, Where It Comes from, How It Sabotages Our Lives by Pia Mellody and J. Keith Miller. Harper San Francisco, 1989.

Audio Cassette

The Price of Nice by John Bradshaw. Bradshaw Cassettes, 1998.

Web Links

www.ola-is.org
www.atdrpats.com/codepend.html
www.drirene.com/boundari.htm

UFO 23: "CANTDOENZA" (SELF-DEFEATING BELIEFS)

While most of us tend to ignore our "casual" thoughts and choice of words, the ways that they shape and influence us go deeper than we know. The language we use and the places we go in our heads when we're troubled or stressed can actually set us up to do things that keep us from getting fit. For example, consider these statements (do you say or think these things?):

- Working out (or dieting) is a pain in the neck (or butt).
- I don't have any discipline—I'm not motivated to get in shape.
- I'm sick and tired of _____ (fill in the blank), but it's something I can't control.
- Because of my genes, I *know* that I'll always be fat and out of shape.

Recommendations

1. Self-defeating beliefs can be overcome with energy work. See Chapter Seven to learn how energy therapy can be used.
2. Be conscious of what you dwell on and the words that you typically choose. Ask a friend to take notice of the ways you put yourself down. Have him or her remind you not to use self-critical words.

Books

Get Out of Your Own Way: Overcoming Self-Defeating Behavior by Mark Goulston, M.D., and Philip Goldberg. Perigee, 1996.

Your Body Believes Every Word You Say by Barbara Hoberman Levine. Aslan Publishing, 1991.

The HeartMath Solution: The Institute of HeartMath's Revolutionary Program for Engaging the Power of the Heart's Intelligence by Doc Lew Childre, Howard Martin, and Donna Beech (Contributor). Harper San Francisco, 2000.

Web Links

www.heartmath.org
www.heartmath.com

For information on energy therapy treatments:

www.emofree.com
www.tftrx.com
www.psychinnovations.com
www.energypsych.com

UFO 24: NEGATIVE ASSOCIATIONS WITH EXERCISE

I've found that for every five people I see who say they don't like to work out, four of them say that it stems from a painful experience in their youth. Examples are being chosen last when friends were picking teams and performing poorly or suffering an injury when playing a sport. Traumatic gym class memories also can cause this UFO, which often makes people feel phobic about working out or joining a gym.

Recommendations

1. Try working out in places, or with people, you enjoy. Examples of places to exercise are the beach or a scenic route, or a river, pond, or lake where you can swim, row a boat, or canoe.
2. Remember, your present experiences don't have to reflect your past. You might be surprised by what you are able to do with a little support.

Books

When Working Out Isn't Working Out: A Mind-Body Guide to Conquering Unidentified Fitness Obstacles by Michael Gerrish. St. Martin's Griffin, 1999.

Web Links

www.active.com
www.nutricise.com

UFO 25: "VICTIMITIS"

People who feel like victims think about life in terms of *shoulds*. For example, they believe people *should* be sensitive to their needs. Or, a nutrition and exercise plan *should* work without any snags. If this sounds like you, it's time to reconsider your point of view. There are no *shoulds* when it comes to getting in shape and losing weight.

Here are some common *shoulds* that can keep you from reaching your fitness goals:

- I *shouldn't* have to work so hard to lose this extra weight.
- My trainer *should've* encouraged me to stick with my routine.
- My nutritionist *should've* given me more ideas about what to eat.

Recommendations

1. Self-defeating behavior often stems from conditioned beliefs—beliefs that are often called rackets, i.e., stories that keep us stuck. Even if

your old patterns don't relate to alcohol use, Al-Alon can provide insight into conquering self-imposed blocks.

2. Consider getting some counseling to let go of false beliefs. Behavior and cognitive therapy may provide the help you need.

Books

Stand Up for Your Life: Develop the Courage, Confidence, and Character to Fulfill Your Greatest Potential by Cheryl Richardson. Free Press, 2002.

Web Links

www.al-anon.alateen.org
www.ola-is.org

UFO 26: IMPROPER EXERCISE TECHNIQUE

Review the exercise guidelines in Chapters Three and Four.

Books

When Working Out Isn't Working Out: A Mind-Body Guide to Conquering Unidentified Fitness Obstacles by Michael Gerrish. St. Martin's Griffin, 1999.

Web Links

www.exerciseplus.com

UFO 27: OVERTRAINING

If you're doing more than your body really needs to achieve your goals, you may be slowing your progress and/or limiting your success. To determine if you're overtraining, use the following as a guide.

You're probably overtraining if you:

- Train seven days a week
- Perform cardiovascular exercise for sixty minutes or more
- Consistently exceed your target heart rate when you train
- Often train the same muscle groups without a day of rest

- Spend more than sixty minutes using machines or lifting weights
- Consistently train when you're injured or ill (or have gone a long time without food)
- Don't allow time to recover when going from one workout to the next

Recommendation

Review the exercise guidelines in Chapters Three and Four. When you work out, it's important to bear in mind that less is more. Remember, it's not how much you do, it's how you *do* what you do!

Books

When Working Out Isn't Working Out: A Mind-Body Guide to Conquering Unidentified Fitness Obstacles by Michael Gerrish. St. Martin's Griffin, 1999.

A Practical Approach to Strength Training by Matt Brzycki. McGraw-Hill/NTC, 1995.

UFO 28: UNDERTRAINING

In general, if you're not exercising with weights at least twice a week, you're probably not working out enough to achieve appreciable gains. Moreover, if you normally do fewer reps than you're capable of, your effort may not be intense enough to ensure a good result. The same goes for training aerobically at a level that is too low, i.e., on a scale of one to five, your perceived exertion is two.

Undertraining often results from the following common mistakes:

- Failing to train to "failure" (ending each set at a random point)
- Consistently being unfocused (being distracted when you work out)
- Consistently resting too long between each set of an exercise

Recommendations

Use the following guidelines to revise the way you train:

1. Use the perceived exertion scale to adjust how hard you train. Please see page 99 for more about how to use this scale.
2. Always train to failure when you're working with weights or machines (this means doing as many reps as you can with perfect form).

3. Do a weight training workout at least two times a week.
4. Do an aerobic workout at least three times a week.

Books

A Practical Approach to Strength Training by Matt Brzycki. McGraw-Hill/NTC, 1995.

UFO 29: EXERCISE ADDICTION

Exercise addiction often takes a tremendous toll, from weakening one's immune system to injuring tendons, muscles, and joints. It can also damage relationships and cause problems at work or at home. This problem can stem from obsessive-compulsive disorder or low self-esteem.

Are you addicted to exercise ? Consider the following signs:

- When you have to miss a workout, you feel guilty, annoyed, or depressed.
- You exercise even when injured, ill, fatigued, or extremely sore.
- The better you look, the more you find parts of your body that need to be "fixed."
- Whenever you miss a workout, you work out twice as much the next day.
- Your body is more important to you than your family, friends, and work.

If you can relate to these statements, you should seek professional help.

Recommendations
1. Do a reality check: Is your behavior paying off? Do you feel energized when you exercise? Have you increased your endurance and strength? Has all your extra work in the gym been worth the results you've achieved? If your answer to even one of these questions is no, it's time for a change. Remember, doing *less* exercise will actually help you *more*.
2. Use meditation or counseling to get symptoms under control.

Books

Hooked on Exercise: How to Understand and Manage Exercise Addiction by Rebecca Prussin, M.D., Philip Harvey, Ph.D., and Theresa Foy DiGeronimo. Simon & Schuster, 1992.

Web Links
www.rrca.org/publicat/addict.html

UFO 30: "EGOMENTIA" (EGO-RELATED ISSUES)

How can your ego keep you from achieving your fitness goals? In more ways than you might imagine, from prompting the use of dangerous drugs to inciting the use of extremely heavy weights with poor technique. Add to the list that it causes appearance obsession (and irritates folks!), and it's easy to see how a wounded or overblown ego can thwart your success.

Recommendations

1. Consider that there may actually be an underlying cause, such as emotional conflicts that relate to poor self-esteem. To get to the root of your problem, consider enlisting professional help.
2. Don't buy into the message we typically get from magazines. Try to step back and remind yourself that ideals are impractical goals.
3. Take a break from the magazines and don't watch so much TV! Remember, each time you see someone you imagine to be ideal, the message you're getting is, "What you see is what you should try to achieve."
4. Find some healthy role models you can relate to, trust, and respect. Often our idols only achieve the appearance of great success, i.e., they change how they look (through questionable means) to mask how they feel. Don't let yourself be fooled by this. Choose your role models with care.

UFO 31: SNACK AMNESIA

Once a nutritionist asked me what I ate during an average day. I recall telling her that most of the time I didn't eat much between meals. But when she had me write down what I ate every day, I received quite a shock. As it turned out, I was typically eating quite a bit more than I thought. I learned that, like many people, I was "grazing" throughout the day.

This wake-up call made me much more aware of what, when, and where I eat. Now I encourage my clients to pay more attention to what *they* eat, mainly by having them keep a log to record everything they consume. It helps them to see more clearly how their choices affect their success.

Recommendation

Record (in a log or journal) what you eat every day for a week. Record the time of day, the food you consume, and your thoughts during the day (don't change the way you normally eat or you won't get an honest result). During the following week, start looking for patterns that keep playing out (continue to keep your food log, being as clear and detailed as you can). Continue using this log as a tool to assess and adjust how you eat. By working with it, you'll discover what really prevents you from losing weight.

UFO 32: IRRITABLE BOWEL SYNDROME (IBS)

It's believed that five million Americans currently suffer from IBS. Symptoms include diarrhea or constipation (sometimes both), as well as abnormal bowel function, intense stomach cramps, and excessive gas.

Recommendations

1. A high-fiber diet is critical to conquering IBS. Metamucil and Citra-Max supplements can also provide relief.
2. Rule out other disorders with appropriate medical tests. To determine if there is bleeding, a lab may need to examine your stools. To examine the large intestine, an enema test may be required.
3. Remember to ask your doctor about new drugs for IBS.
4. Find an IBS support group in your area (or online).
5. Consider hypnosis or counseling to reduce your level of stress.

Books

Eating for IBS: 175 Delicious, Nutritious, Low-Fat, Low-Residue Recipes to Stabilize the Touchiest Tummy by Heather Van Vorous. Marlowe & Co., 2000.

Breaking the Bonds of Irritable Bowel Syndrome: A Psychological Approach to Regaining Control of Your Life by Barbara Bradley Bolen, Ph.D., and W. Grant Thompson. New Harbinger, 2000.

25 Natural Ways to Relieve Irritable Bowel Syndrome: A Mind-Body Approach to Well-Being by James Scala. McGraw-Hill/NTC, 2000.

www.panix.com/~ibs
www.medhelp.org/healthtopics/ibs.html

Self-help groups:

www.ibsgroup.org (in Canada)
www.iffgd.org

UFO 33: DIET MISCONCEPTIONS

If you typically get your diet advice from friends or magazines, there's a pretty good chance you're putting your faith in advice that is steering you wrong.

Examples of misconceptions are that supplements pose no risk, most diet foods are "healthy," and particular foods burn fat. To discover *your* misconceptions, review the advice in Chapter Six.

Recommendation
Remember that studies are often skewed to support a company's claims. For example, if you see an ad for a weight-loss drug in a magazine, don't be fooled by the "research" citing fair and impartial results. If something sounds too good to be true, assume that it probably is.

Books
Eating Well for Optimum Health: The Essential Guide to Food, Diet, and Nutrition by Andrew Weil, M.D. Knopf, 2000.

The Diet Cure: The 8-Step Program to Rebalance Your Body Chemistry and End Food Cravings, Weight Problems, and Mood Swings—Now by Julia Ross. Penguin USA, 2000.

Prescription for Nutritional Healing: A Practical A to Z Reference to Drug-Free Remedies Using Vitamins, Minerals, Herbs & Food Supplements, 3rd ed., by Phyllis A. Balch, C.N.C., and James F. Balch, M.D. Avery, 2000.

Web Links
www.cyberdiet.com
www.navigator.tufts.edu
www.nutrition.gov/home/index.php3

UFO 34: INSULIN INSTABILITY

Insulin instability is a popular topic these days, as evidenced by the appeal of the Atkins diet and the Zone. If you are insulin sensitive, you should avoid high-glycemic foods (they are likely to cause your blood sugar level to spike and then to crash). This will decrease the rate at which your body will burn fat. It will also rob you of energy (making you less apt to go to the gym).

Recommendations

1. Adjust your balance of protein, fat, and carbohydrates (see Chapter Six). I believe most people would do well to reduce their intake of carbs, but I'm not convinced that the optimum balance of carbs is 40 percent. To start, I suggest your carb intake be closer to 50 percent. See Chapter Six, Plan B (page 193) to learn how this works.
2. Increase your daily intake of fatty acids (omega-3). They will stabilize your blood sugar and help you eliminate "unhealthy" fat. Barlean's flaxseed capsules are an excellent source of omega-3, as are OmegaBrite capsules (www.omegabrite.com).
3. If your energy swings are severe when you consume starchy or sugary foods, you're probably insulin sensitive and should avoid high-glycemic foods. To determine if you are really insulin sensitive, try this test: avoid the foods that are listed in the next section for one week. Keep a log to record how you feel and your weight at the end of the week. Use the log to assess your results and adjust what you eat each day.

High-Glycemic Foods

High-glycemic foods are absorbed very quickly into your blood, triggering blood sugar swings that can make you feel weak and/or fatigued. (From *Mastering the Zone* by Barry Sears, Ph.D.)

- *Extremely High:* puffed rice, cornflakes, millet, instant rice, instant potato, French bread, cooked parsnips, baked potato, cooked carrots, fava beans, white bread, foods containing simple sugars (maltose, glucose, and honey)
- *High:* wheat bread, Grape-Nuts cereal, tortilla chips, shredded wheat, muesli, rye bread, brown rice, oats, sweet corn, white rice, mashed potato, boiled potato, apricots, raisins, bananas, papaya, mango, corn chips, candy, crackers, cookies, pastry, low-fat ice cream

- *Moderately High:* buckwheat, bran cereal, spaghetti, yams, sweet potato, green peas, baked beans, kidney beans, fruit cocktail, grapefruit juice, orange juice, pineapple juice, canned pears, grapes, potato chips, sponge cake

Books

Syndrome X: Managing Insulin Resistance by Deborah S. Romaine, Jennifer B. Marks, M.D., and Glenn S. Rothfeld, M.D. Harper Mass Market Paperbacks, 2000.

Protein Power by Michael Eades, M.D., and Mary Dan Eades. Bantam Doubleday Dell, 1999.

Mastering the Zone by Barry Sears, Ph.D. HarperCollins, 1997.

The Carbohydrate Addict's Diet: The Lifelong Solution to Yo-Yo Dieting by Dr. Rachael F. Heller and Dr. Richard F. Heller. Signet, 1993.

Web Links

www.zoneperfect.com/site/content/index.asp

UFO 35: AMINO ACID DEFICIENCY

Amino acids are often called our body's "building blocks." From tissue repair and cell building to fighting illness and building strength, amino acids are critical to maintaining optimum health. They also help stabilize blood sugar levels and oxygenate the blood.

An amino acid deficiency can be confirmed by testing your blood. If you do have a deficiency, various supplements can be prescribed, depending on what your symptoms are and what blood tests reveal. For example, if you have a virus, it may be a sign that you lack lysine. If you have candidiasis, it may mean that you need taurine.

If you have this type of deficiency, you may be sick for long stretches of time and may also feel depleted, as if your body is running on fumes. You may also find it hard to increase muscle mass and reduce body fat.

Recommendations

1. An amino acid deficiency can be confirmed by a blood test. The results will help your doctor determine exactly what you need, as hit-or-miss supplement choices can make an imbalance even worse.

2. Ask about taking a customized amino acid blend. Your doctor can assess the specific types your body needs and arrange for a supplement company to combine them in the right dose.
3. Find out if you might be deficient due to problems you haven't explored: for example, leaky gut syndrome, hypochlorhydria, or IBS (irritable bowel syndrome).

Books

The Amino Revolution by Robert Erdmann and Meirion Jones. Fireside, 1989.

Amino Acids in Therapy by Leon Chaitow. Inner Traditions Intl. Ltd., 1985.

Amino Acid Metabolism and Therapy in Health and Nutritional Disease by Luc A. Cynober (Ed.). CRC Press, 1995.

Web Links

www.realtime.net/anr/aminoacd.html
www.healingwithnutrition.com/aminoacid.html

UFO 36: IMPROPER FOOD COMBINING

Because we require different enzymes to digest different types of foods, there are some combinations that many of us would do very well to avoid. For example, fruits and vegetables should not be combined during a meal, as the enzymes we require to break them down are not the same.

High-carbohydrate foods, such as rice, potatoes, pasta, and bread, require an *alkaline* medium to be broken down and fully absorbed. Conversely, an *acid* medium is required for high-protein foods. So while the old adage "You are what you eat" may seem to make pretty good sense, perhaps a more accurate statement is "You are what you absorb."

Recommendations

1. Choose foods from the meat, grain, and dairy groups during the latter half of the day.
2. Avoid eating fruits and vegetables together at any meal.
3. Do not consume "pure" fats, such as cream and butter, with starchy foods.
4. Avoid eating highly acidic foods with those that are high in starch. Examples of highly acidic foods are vinegar and citrus fruit.

5. In general, avoid eating high-protein foods with foods that are high in starch.

Books

Fit for Life 2 by Harvey Diamond and Marilyn Diamond. Warner Books, 1987.

The Schwarzbein Principle: The Truth About Losing Weight, Being Healthy, and Feeling Younger by Diana Schwarzbein. Health Communications, 1999.

Food Combining: A Step-by-Step Guide by Kathryn Marsden. Element Books Limited, 1999.

Web Links

www.internethealthlibrary.com/dietandlifestyle/food_combining.htm
http://weightloss.about.com/cs/foodcombining
www.ayurveda.com/info/foodcomb.htm

UFO 37: IMPROPER USE OF SUPPLEMENTS

I often wince when people ask, "What supplements should I take?" This is because it's rare that anyone likes what I have to say: "It's hard for me to be certain because everyone has different needs." In addition, individual needs can vary from week to week. Moreover, I don't think it's wise to base what you take on the RDA (recommended daily allowance), as these guidelines are much too broad to account for specific personal needs.

Recommendations

1. Research computerized diet logs or those on a handheld device. (See the Web Links.) These logs will give you a general idea of the nutrients you require.
2. Get your diet analyzed at a website (free of charge). To learn exactly how this works, go to www.ag.uiuc.edu/~food-lab/nat.
3. Consult a medical doctor with an alternative medicine bent. Many alternative healers have great faith in their expertise, oftentimes to the point where they're quite cavalier about what they prescribe. The result is that they often fail to consider important facts: For example, can certain supplements counteract the effects of a drug? Could the supplements worsen a health condition that neither you nor the healer

even know exists? While many alternative healers are quite good at what they do, it's best to proceed with caution (and see your medical doctor first).

4. Consult a nutritionist who is well informed about supplement use.

Books

Prescription for Nutritional Healing: A Practical A to Z Reference to Drug-Free Remedies Using Vitamins, Minerals, Herbs & Food Supplements, 3rd ed., by Phyllis A. Balch, C.N.C., and James F. Balch, M.D. Avery, 2000.

The PDR Family Guide to Nutritional Supplements: An Authoritative A–to–Z Guide to the 100 Most Popular Nutritional Therapies and Nutraceuticals. Ballantine Books, 2001.

An Evaluation of Popular Fitness-Enhancing Supplements by Neal Spruce and Alan Titchenal. Evergreen Communications, 2001.

Web Links

www.crnusa.org/1newsreleases.html
http://ods.od.nih.gov/databases/ibids.html
http://dmoz.org/health/nutrition/nutrients_in_foods/vitamins_and_minerals

To learn about diet logs:

www.iddiet.com
www.doithome.com
www.dietpower.com
http://dmoz.org/shopping/health/weight_loss/software

Creatine is a supplement used to enhance endurance and strength. Properly used, it creates a reserve of energy in muscle cells. To learn about creatine supplements:

www.sportsci.org/traintech/creatine/rbk.html
www.quackwatch.com/01quackeryrelatedtopics/dsh/creatine.html
www.mdausa.org/research/creatine.html

Ephedra is a stimulant that is a popular weight loss aid. Derived from the ephedra plant, it is also called *Ma Huang*. To learn about ephedra:

www.ephedrafacts.com
www.recalledproduct.com/recalledephedra
www.ephedrine-ephedra.com/pages/ephedrine_side_effects.html

UFO 38: "HEAVY BAGGAGE SYNDROME" (UNRESOLVED EMOTIONAL ISSUES)

Of course, we all have our "issues," but perhaps you have more than your share? Examples of unresolved issues are a history of being abused, anger toward family members, and resentment toward critical peers. Pent-up emotional baggage can actually keep you from getting in shape, for example, by causing you to gain weight to "shield" yourself from abuse.

Recommendations
1. See Chapter Seven for treatments to address your specific needs.
2. Consider seeing a counselor to reveal and heal old wounds. Exposing the root of emotional blocks can help you physically, too.

Books

Breaking Free from Anger: Overcoming Unresolved Resentment, Overwhelming Emotions, and Angry Reactions by Neil T. Anderson and Rich Miller. Harvest House Publishers, Inc., 2002.

Healing the Shame That Binds You by John E. Bradshaw. Health Communications, 1988.

Breaking the Power: Of Unmet Needs, Unhealed Hurts, Unresolved Issues in Your Life by Liberty Savard. Bridge-Logos Publishers, 1997.

UFO 39: "QUICKFIXIA NERVOSA" (ERRATIC DIET HISTORY)

If the thought of a brand-new diet makes you excited to give it a try, you've probably tried a lot of them, many of which have failed to work. Even the ones that did work probably didn't have lasting results, leaving you feeling hopeless, disappointed, and very confused. To help put an end to this saga, give some thought to the following points.

Recommendations

1. To discover what type of plan is best for you, see Chapter Six.
2. See a nutritionist for a plan that's tailored to meet your needs.
3. A diet won't work unless you work on the things that will make it work! Translation: Address your UFOs or your diet is doomed to fail.
4. Don't consume foods you're allergic to or that trigger energy swings.

Books

The Diet Cure: The 8-Step Program to Rebalance Your Body Chemistry and End Food Cravings, Weight Problems, and Mood Swings—Now by Julia Ross. Penguin USA, 2000.

The Yo-Yo Diet Syndrome: How to Heal and Stabilize Your Appetite and Weight by Doreen Virtue. Hay House, 1997.

Web Links

http://weightloss.about.com/cs/yoyodieting
www.ahealthyme.com/topic/yoyodieting

UFO 40: SELF-SABOTAGE

When it comes to finding time to work out and successfully losing weight, self-sabotage is a problem that can be difficult to resolve. Examples are going to places where you'll be tempted by fattening foods or trying to do too much the first few times you go to the gym.

Recommendations

1. Identify how your fears play out and affect the way you behave. For example, do you feel vulnerable when you think about losing weight? Does a fear of being "noticed" make you sabotage your success? Keeping a journal will help you reveal any patterns that keep you stuck.
2. Consider your true motivation for pursuing your physical goals. For example, are you dieting to appease a critical spouse? Make sure that your goals are aligned with what makes sense and is best for *you*.

Books

Extreme Success by Rich Fettke. Fireside, 2002.

Freedom from Self-Sabotage: The Intelligent Reader's Guide to Success and Self-Fulfillment by Peter A. Michaelson. Prospect Books, 1999.

What's Your Sabotage? by Alyce P. Cornyn-Selby. Beynch Press Publishing Co., 2000.

UFO 41: SLEEP APNEA

Sleep apnea is a problem that too often goes undiagnosed. Irregular, labored breathing is the most commonly cited concern, the primary consequence being the prevention of quality sleep. If you suffer from this condition, people have probably said that you snore and may have observed that your breathing often stops when you're asleep. Other symptoms are allergies, sinus pain, and frequent colds.

Sleep apnea can prevent you from getting in shape in the following ways:

- It robs your blood of oxygen, which can lead to daytime fatigue.
- It can result in sleep debt, which if ongoing and severe can make you fatigue more quickly when your body is under stress.

Recommendations

1. To ensure that your airway is open, elevate the head of your bed. Use extra pillows or pads to keep your head and torso raised.
2. Stay away from alcohol or drugs that can sedate. Studies show that alcohol usually makes sleep apnea *worse*.
3. To breathe with greater ease, sleep on your side as opposed to your back.
4. *Do not smoke*, particularly before you go to bed. Smoking increases the frequency and severity of labored breaths.
5. Try adhesive nose strips or antisnoring aids.
6. If your symptoms are clearly chronic and have been diagnosed as severe, a continuous positive air pressure (CPAP) device should give relief. It will help to keep your throat open and get more oxygen into your blood.
7. Get a dental appliance you can wear while you're asleep. It will move your tongue and jaw forward, which will help to open your throat.
8. Consider corrective surgery if your problem is severe. You may have to enlarge your air passage so you can breathe comfortably when you sleep.

Books

Snoring and Sleep Apnea: Sleep Well, Feel Better, 3rd ed., by Ralph Pascualy, M.D. Demos Medical Publishing, 2000.

Stop the Snoring! by Ralph Schoenstein and Yosef Krespi. Warner Books, 1997.

Web Links

www.sleepquest.com

UFO 42: DELAYED SLEEP PHASE SYNDROME (DSPS)

If you like to rise late in the morning and go to bed very late at night, it may be because, compared to the norm, your sleep phase is delayed. The symptoms are waking and rising late in the morning or afternoon and going to bed unusually late, i.e., after 2 A.M. Other symptoms are brain fog, poor concentration, and memory loss, as well as feeling extremely fatigued long after an early rise.

Recommendations

1. *Chronotherapy.* To reset your clock, rise one hour earlier every day. For example, to rise at 6 A.M. (if you normally wake at noon), set your alarm for 11 A.M. on day 1 and get right out of bed. Set it for 10 A.M. on day 2 and keep moving it back every day. The goal is to rise feeling rested (every day!) at 6 A.M.
2. *Full-spectrum bright-light therapy.* Bright light has been used with great success to modify patterns of sleep. (You would normally turn the light on just before you plan to rise.) Consult a sleep/wake specialist for specific treatment advice.

Books

The Circadian Prescription by Sidney MacDonald, M.D., and Karen Baar. Perigee, 2001.

Web Links

www.sleepdisorderchannel.net/dsps
http://sleepdisorders.about.com/cs/dsps
www.apollolight.com/biological_clock.html

UFO 43: ADVANCED SLEEP PHASE SYNDROME (ASPS)

Advanced sleep phase syndrome (ASPS) is fairly rare but seems to occur more often in people over age sixty-five. Symptoms are:

- Falling asleep very early, for example, before 8 P.M.
- Waking up well before you plan to rise and start your day
- Feeling extremely tired when staying up past 8 P.M.
- Marital difficulties, due to schedules that conflict
- Abusing sleep medication, alcohol, or other drugs

Recommendations

1. *Chronotherapy.* Go to bed one hour later every day to reset your clock. For example, if you normally fall asleep at 8 P.M., on day 1 (no matter how tired you are) go to bed at 9 P.M. Then, on day 2, plan to go to bed at 10 P.M.
2. *Full-spectrum bright-light therapy.* Bright light has been used with great success to modify patterns of sleep. (You would normally turn the light on just before you plan to rise.) Consult a sleep/wake specialist for specific treatment advice.

Books

The Circadian Prescription by Sidney MacDonald, M.D., and Karen Baar. Perigee, 2001.

Web Links

www.stanford.edu/~dement/advanced.html
www.apollolight.com/page3.html

UFO 44: RESTLESS LEG SYNDROME (RLS)

If you have a restless leg problem, you're probably not getting quality sleep, which can limit your energy level, strength, and stamina when you train. Symptoms are restless or twitchy legs (before or while you're asleep) and feeling compelled to move or shake your legs while lying in bed. These symptoms are often relieved by stretching your legs or walking around. Getting massaged, working out, or taking a bath can help as well.

Recommendations

1. If you're taking a drug, try a new type or take a different dose. Some studies show that Prozac can make restless leg symptoms worse. Ask your doctor what types of drugs can exacerbate RLS. In addition, ask what options you have for changing your drug or dose.
2. Ask your doctor about the drugs that are used for RLS. Carbidopa-levodopa (Sinemet) is often prescribed, as well as anticonvulsants, opioids, and Klonopin.
3. A folic acid supplement may provide additional help. According to many homeopaths, it helps calm restless legs.
4. Avoid consuming caffeine, especially after 6 P.M.

Books

Sleep Thief: Restless Legs Syndrome by Virginia N. Wilson, David Buchholz, and Arthur S. Walters. Galaxy Books, Inc., 1996.

Web Links

http://members.aol.com/biobrite/sleep
www.rls.org

UFO 45: WORK ADDICTION

These days it seems that many of us mistake our jobs for a life and are too busy, driven, or stressed to see the forest for the trees. If this means you, and you don't start seeing the forest fairly soon, there's a very good chance that you'll end up sick or neglecting your family and friends.

The irony is that when you work too much and skimp on sleep, it lowers your energy level, making you more apt to do poor work! Putting this into perspective may be the key to reversing this trend.

Recommendations

1. Don't take your work to bed, and get at least eight solid hours of sleep.
2. Don't let too much time go by without having something to eat. If you're a workaholic, there's a good chance that you're skipping meals, so plan to bring food to the office or have it delivered to you each day.

Also, avoid eating junk food, such as pizza, donuts, and sweets. Stick to healthier snacks, such as vegetables, fruit, and unsalted nuts.

3. Reserve weekends for your family and resolve not to talk about work.
4. Work on only one thing at a time—stop juggling so many balls!

Books

The Man Who Mistook His Job for a Life: A Chronic Overachiever Finds the Way Home by Jonathon Lazear. Crown, 2001.

Chained to the Desk: A Guidebook for Workaholics, Their Partners and Children, and the Clinicians Who Treat Them by Bryan E. Robinson, Ph.D. New York University Press, 2001.

Work Addiction: Hidden Legacies of Adult Children by Bryan E. Robinson, Ph.D. Health Communications, 1989.

Web Links

http://people.ne.mediaone.net/wa2/#wso
http://directory.google.com/top/society/work/workaholism/support_groups

Support groups:

www.mlode.com/~ra/ra2/workaholism.htm

UFO 46: POOR LIFE/TIME MANAGEMENT

Clearly, of all the excuses I hear from people who don't work out, the one that I hear most often is "I just don't have the time." To me what this *really* means is that you have put less important things first. To prove my point, imagine you're told you must exercise or you'll *die*. Do you think hearing this might change your view about whether you have enough time? (If your answer is no, you can stop reading here—you're clearly beyond my help!) So the problem is *not* that you don't have time—it's where your priorities lie. And there shouldn't be many priorities that take precedence over your health.

Recommendations

1. Identify all the *real* reasons that you don't have time to work out. Could it be that you've buried yourself in work to avoid facing something you fear? Do you have marital problems, issues with money, or

problems at work? Think about why you're so busy; do you *really* not have any choice?

2. Instead of the elevator (or escalator), take the stairs. Can you think of any other ways to exercise during the day? How about calling clients on your cell phone while taking a walk? Or doing push-ups in your office using your desk or chair as a prop? Use your imagination—you'll be surprised by what you can do.

3. Spend quality time with your kids and get some exercise at the same time. Join them for a street hockey game, bike ride, or hike in the woods. Instead of just watching your kids run around, ask them if you can play, too!

Books

Take Time for Your Life: A Personal Coach's 7-Step Program for Creating the Life You Want by Cheryl Richardson. Broadway Books, 1998.

Time Management from the Inside Out: The Foolproof System for Taking Control of Your Schedule and Your Life by Julie Morgenstern. Henry Holt, 2000.

Fitting in Fitness: Hundreds of Simple Ways to Put More Physical Activity Into Your Life by the American Heart Association. Times Books, 1997.

UFO 47: OSTEOPOROSIS

If you have osteoporosis, you have brittle or fragile bones. If you do, and it goes untreated, you are susceptible to a break, which is likely to involve areas such as your spine, hips, feet, or wrists. Women account for 80 percent of those with this disease, and one out of every two women over fifty is at risk.

Osteoporosis is mainly caused by a decrease in bone mass, which can often result in hip fractures, severe back pain, and loss of height.

Recommendations

1. Increase your intake of foods that are rich in calcium and vitamin D. Examples are green leafy vegetables, yogurt, milk, fish oil, and eggs.

2. Perform weight-bearing exercise at least three times a week. Research shows that weight training is ideal for strengthening bones.

3. Limit your alcohol intake, and if you smoke, resolve to quit.

4. Be sure to take a bone density test, preferably once a year. It will measure your rate of bone loss and reveal where bones are weak.

5. Ask your physician about taking drugs to increase the strength of your bones. Estrogen, calcitonin, and alendronate are often prescribed, but new drugs may be available (ask your doctor for advice).

Books

The Bone Density Diet: 6 Weeks to a Strong Body and Mind by George J. Kessler DO PC, and Colleen Kapklein (Contributor). Ballantine Books, 2000.

Osteoporosis Cure: Reverse the Crippling Effects with New Treatment by Harris H. McIlwain and Debra Fulghum Bruce. Avon, 1998.

Strong Women, Strong Bones: Everything You Need to Know to Prevent, Treat, and Beat Osteoporosis by Miriam E. Nelson and Sarah Wernick. Perigee, 2001.

Web Links

www.nof.org
www.strongwomen.com
www.osteo.org
www.learn-about-osteoporosis.com

UFO 48: UNRECOGNIZED SIDE EFFECTS (PRESCRIPTION AND OVER-THE-COUNTER DRUGS)

Overlooked drug interactions and side effects can be UFOs. Symptoms that often are overlooked are insomnia and fatigue, as well as weight gain, fluid retention, depression, and memory loss. If you're taking a drug and you're not feeling right, *do not* be resigned to your fate! Talk to your doctor about how you feel and make the appropriate change.

Recommendations

1. The more different drugs you take, the greater the chance side effects will occur. Be sure to talk to your doctor if you are taking more than one drug.
2. Alert your pharmacist if you're taking hormone replacement drugs. These drugs often increase or decrease the potency of other drugs.
3. Don't disregard any symptoms—tell your doctor how you feel.
4. Read the information you get from your pharmacy with your drug.
5. Don't stop taking a drug without consulting your doctor first.

Books

The PDR Pocket Guide to Prescription Drugs by Robert W. Hogan. Pocket Books, 2002.

The Pill Book by Harold Silverman. Bantam Books, 2000.

Dangerous Drug Interactions by Joe Graedon and Teresa Graedon. St. Martin's Press, 1999.

Web Links

www.torsades.org
www.pdr.net
www.nlm.nih.gov/medlineplus/druginformation.html

UFO 49: ADRENAL BURNOUT

When you're under stress, your adrenal glands can easily be overworked, initially causing an increase in cortisol and DHEA. In the second stage of "burnout," both of these hormones will *decrease*, which can cause frequent urination, fluid retention, and extreme thirst. Other burnout symptoms include hair loss, joint pain, and fatigue, as well as depression, recurring infections, ulcers, and problems with sleep.

Recommendations

1. To find out if you're suffering from burnout, take the adrenal stress index (ASI) test. Ask your doctor for more details about what this test involves.
2. Depending on the circumstance, the following may be prescribed: adrenal glandular, pregnenolone, cortisol, and DHEA. Ginseng and licorice supplements may be recommended too, as well as B-complex, zinc, and vitamins A, C, E, and B_6.
3. Stay away from acidic foods, such as citrus fruits and wine. People with stressed adrenals often don't tolerate these types of food.
4. Choline, coenzyme Q-10, and inositol may be worth a try. Desiccated adrenal supplements and PABA may help as well.
5. Try meditation, yoga, acupuncture, or massage.
6. Ask your doctor if any new drugs have recently been approved.

Books

Tired of Being Tired: Rescue, Repair, Rejuvenate by Jesse Hanley and Nancy Deville. Putnam Publishing Group, 2001.

Web Links

www.healburnout.com/causes2.html

http://myhealth.medformation.com/excerpt.asp?excerptid=638

UFO 50: TOXIC RELATIONSHIP SYNDROME

If your coworkers, family, and friends are often envious of your success or so self-absorbed that they couldn't care less about you or how you feel, it's time to take a good look at how these relationships need to change. Too often we accept less—*far* less—from folks than we truly deserve. Examples are letting a friend discourage your efforts to get in shape or allowing someone to pressure you to consume a fattening food. Often a partner or spouse can be the primary saboteur, for example, by making rude comments about the way you dress or look.

Recommendations

1. Learn how to set stronger boundaries and resolve to keep them firm.
2. Make a clear and firm request for nonjudgmental support.
3. Be willing to give up relationships that hurt you more than they help.
4. Create some affirmations to help strengthen your resolve. Examples are "I will stand up for myself, regardless of what others think," or "I don't have to listen to anyone who doesn't support my growth."
5. Use the Imago process to resolve interpersonal rifts (see the Web Links to find out how this process works).

Books

Co-Dependence: Misunderstood-Mistreated by Anne Wilson Schaef. Harper San Francisco, 1992.

Emotional Blackmail: When the People in Your Life Use Fear, Obligation and Guilt to Manipulate You by Susan Forward and Donna Frazier. HarperCollins, 1998.

Nasty People by Jay Carter. McGraw-Hill/NTC, 1989.

www.imagotherapy.com
www.healthyrelating.com

UFO 51: "ASKAPHOBIA" (FEAR OF ASKING FOR HELP)

The reasons we don't ask for help can range from a fear of appearing weak to thinking we already know everything (or wanting to hide that we don't!). Being too stubborn or shy to ask for help can impede your success, as trying to figure things out by yourself can waste a lot of time. Moreover, asking for help will ensure that you won't get hurt in the gym.

Recommendations

1. Ask and ye shall receive! But if you don't, ask someone else! Wyatt Webb, a therapist, offers this simple but cogent advice:

   - If something isn't working for you, try doing something else.
   - If what you're doing still doesn't work, ask someone for help.
   - If what you're doing still doesn't work, ask someone else for help.

2. The answer to just one question may be the key to a radical change. The advice you get could totally change your perspective on getting in shape, enabling you to attain results that you otherwise wouldn't achieve.

Books

Stand Up for Your Life: Develop the Courage, Confidence, and Character to Fulfill Your Greatest Potential by Cheryl Richardson. Free Press, 2002.

It's Not About the Horse by Wyatt Webb. Hay House, 2002.

UFO 52: "CONNECTAPHOBIA" (FEAR OF INTIMACY)

How can a fear of intimacy prevent you from getting in shape? By making you prone to self-sabotage due to discomfort about being slim. For example, if getting too close to folks is a notion that triggers fear, you may gain weight to make those who would find you attractive stay away.

Recommendations

1. See Chapter Seven to learn how energy work can shift your beliefs.
2. Consider seeing a therapist to determine the cause of your fear. Perhaps an abusive experience that you've suppressed is at the root? Or perhaps your relationship history has involved being hurt or deceived? Whatever the case, it is critical that you express your concerns and fears.

Books

The Dance of Intimacy: A Woman's Guide to Courageous Acts of Change in Key Relationships by Harriet Lerner. HarperCollins, 1990.

Go Away, Come Closer: When What You Need the Most Is What You Fear the Most by Terry Hershey. Hershey & Associates, 1990.

Web Links

http://joy2meu.com
www.nvo.com/fearofintimacy

To learn about energy therapy:

www.emofree.com
www.tftrx.com
www.psychinnovations.com
www.energypsych.com

UFO 53: SLEEP DEBT

Sleep deprivation can harm you in a number of serious ways. When you are sleep deprived, you are more vulnerable to stress, which can manifest through your body, causing pain in your head, back, and neck. In addition, you have less energy for the things that could help you "heal," such as spending more time with your family, eating good food, or working out.

Recommendations

1. Practice good "sleep hygiene," i.e., *plan* to get better sleep. Consider this list of ways to ensure you get all the sleep you need:

   - Listen to peaceful music before, or while, you lie in bed (I suggest you use a timer so your stereo shuts itself off). Or try a relaxation tape (I'm a fan of Brian Weiss).

- Read something (unrelated to current events) while lying in bed. Get yourself lost in a story that evokes relaxing thoughts.
- Always wear something comfortable and be sure your bed has clean sheets.
- Go to bed at the same time every night and develop a sleep routine; for example, take time to meditate, read a book, or take a bath.
- Soundproof your room, wear ear plugs, and make sure doors and windows are closed.
- Don't eat anything heavy for three hours before you retire.
- Restricting your bathroom visits can be a key to better sleep. Remember not to drink too much before you go to bed.
- Save all discussions and arguments for an appropriate time during the day.

2. If you're thinking about taking sleep aids, talk to your medical doctor first. Even some "natural" remedies can have serious ill effects. For example, research has shown that valerian root is not always safe (it can cause side effects such as nausea, headaches, cramps, and restless sleep).
3. Stay away from substances that may stimulate you at night. This includes aspartame, caffeine, and high-glycemic foods.

Books

Say Goodnight to Insomnia by Gregg D. Jacobs and Herbert Benson. Owl Books, 1999.

No More Sleepless Nights, 2nd ed., by Peter Hauri and Shirley Linde. John Wiley & Sons, 1996.

Power Sleep: The Revolutionary Program That Prepares Your Mind for Peak Performance by James B. Maas, Megan L. Wherry, David J. Axelrod, and Barbara R. Hogan. HarperCollins, 1999.

Desperately Seeking Snoozin': The Insomnia Cure from Awake to Zzzzz by John Wiedman. Towering Pines Press, Inc., 1999.

Web Links

www.sleepnet.com
www.getsleep.com
www.remedyfind.com/hc-sleep-disorders.asp

UFO 54: SHADOW BELIEFS

Shadow beliefs can debilitate you, says author Debbie Ford, unless you learn to use them to *support* your personal growth. In a nutshell, Debbie's message is "Gain wisdom from your wounds." By looking at themes that keep playing out repeatedly in your life, you can start to uncover your core beliefs and see how they hold you back.

Shadow beliefs can keep you mired in self-defeating ruts, complaining that life isn't fair and thinking that things will never change. A critical inner voice will often mirror a shadow belief, as well as abusive behavior and bad habits that keep you stuck.

By looking at what upsets or angers you most about someone else, you can get to the root of your shadow beliefs and use them to change your life. For example, if you criticize those who dress in provocative ways, there may be a part of you that would like to wear bolder styles of clothes. Or if you're someone who bristles when people are critical of your work, there may be a part of you that is actually critical of *yourself*.

Recommendations

1. Think about who, or what, you blame for the problems you typically face. Who makes you feel like a victim? What gets you most upset? Do certain things make you angry, sad, resentful, or ashamed?
2. Think about people you envy and the things about them you dislike. What does this say about who you are and how is it linked to your past? Your answer may give you some clues about parts of yourself that you need to embrace.
3. Consider the story you're living right now and how you would like it to change. Then write down your story so that the details become more clear.
4. Compose an all-new story that describes how your life would change. Create an ideal situation—what would your best-case scenario be? How would you have to change yourself to make this story true?

Books

The Dark Side of the Light Chasers: Reclaiming Your Power, Creativity, Brilliance, and Dreams by Debbie Ford. Riverhead Books, 1999.

The Secret of the Shadow: The Power of Owning Your Whole Story by Debbie Ford. Harper San Francisco, 2001.

http://fordsisters.com/darkside.html
www.debbieford.com

UFO 55: EXERCISE MISCONCEPTIONS

Which of the following exercise misconceptions do you have?

1. The longer you train, the better the gain (two hours are better than one).
2. Unless you feel a lot of pain, you won't achieve much gain.
3. If you build yourself up and stop working out, your muscles will turn to fat.
4. Do lots of leg lifts, sit-ups, crunches, and twists to spot reduce.
5. In order to build more muscle, use free weights instead of machines.
6. Perform explosive movements to increase your muscular gains (to stimulate fast-twitch fibers, it's important to exercise fast).
7. You'll lose less weight when you train with weights because muscle weighs more than fat.
8. Using a heavy weight is more important than using good form.
9. Some areas, such as abdominals, need a lot more reps and sets.
10. To increase fat loss, low-intensity exercise is the key.

Recommendations

1. Be wary of advice you get from friends and magazines. Don't trust any new findings until they've stood the test of time.
2. It's not what you do that matters most, it's how you *do* what you do. Concentrate on refining your form and making each movement count. Make sure you always move in a way that is fluid, slow, and controlled.
3. Limit the number of sets of each exercise to two or three. To do any more is overkill and won't improve your gains.
4. Limit your reps (in general, you should "fail" between six and twelve).
5. If spot reducing really worked, gum chewers would have thin jaws! Don't buy into this fallacy. It will only waste your time.

Books

Health & Fitness Excellence: The Comprehensive Action Plan by Robert K. Cooper. Houghton Mifflin, 1989.

Fitness for Dummies by Suzanne Scholsberg and Liz Neporent. IDG Books, 1996.

UFO 56: PERFECTIONISM

Perfectionists are so afraid to fail that they rarely succeed. For example, they will procrastinate to avoid doing subpar work or won't start a project unless they think they can do a perfect job. This makes perfectionists underachieve, which lowers their self-esteem.

Perfectionists often suffer from eating disorders and panic attacks, as well as depression, migraines, self-sabotage, and image concerns.

Recommendations

1. Perfectionism can make you do a lot of imperfect things, like putting things off, exercising too much, or starving yourself to lose weight. Realizing that this is true can be a key to changing your fate.
2. See Chapter Seven for treatments and affirmations that may help. Examples of affirmations are "I'm doing the best I can," and "I accept myself, although I have made (and will make) mistakes."

Books

Too Perfect—When Being in Control Gets Out of Control by Allan E. Mallinger, M.D., and Jeannette DeWyze. Clarkson Potter, 1992.

Never Good Enough: How to Use Perfectionism to Your Advantage Without Ruining Your Life by Monica Ramirez Basco, Ph.D. Touchstone Books, 2000.

The Care and Feeding of Perfectionists by Cynthia Curnan. North Star Publications Inc., 1999.

Web Links

www.nexus.edu.au/teachstud/gat/peters.htm
www.coping.org/growth/perfect.htm

Perfectionist test:

www.psychtests.com/tests/personality/perfectionism.html

UFO 57: HYPOGLYCEMIA

If you are hypoglycemic, your blood sugar level is often low (less than 45 milligrams per deciliter of blood). Symptoms are dizziness, hunger, irritability, and pale skin, as well as shakiness, sweating, and tingling sensations around the mouth. Other symptoms are headaches, marked weight gain, and inadequate sleep.

Some experts feel that this problem is largely underdiagnosed and claim that conventional tests can't really disprove that this problem exists. So even if tests reveal your blood sugar level is in the right range, your doctor may still suggest you pay more attention to what you eat.

Recommendations

1. Glucagon may help to keep your blood sugar swings at bay. Ask your doctor if glucagon is an option in your case.
2. Eat smaller meals more often so you won't have blood sugar swings. Four to eight small meals a day are what most doctors recommend, consisting mostly of foods that take a longer time to digest. Examples are foods high in protein or low-glycemic carbs.
3. Beware of dextrose, maltose, sucrose, sorbital, and caffeine.
4. Stay away from soda, Gatorade, juice, and sugary drinks.

Books

Beating the Blood Sugar Blues by Thomas A. Lincoln and John A. Eaddy. McGraw-Hill Professional Publishing, 2001.

The Low Blood Sugar Cookbook: Sugarless Cooking for Everyone by Patricia Krimmel and Edward A. Krimmel. Franklin Publishers, 1992.

Carlton Fredericks' New Low Blood Sugar and You by Carlton Fredericks. Perigee, 1985.

Web Links

http://hypoglycemia.itgo.com
www.healthlinkusa.com/hypoglycemia.htm
www.nlm.nih.gov/medlineplus/hypoglycemia.html
http://healthed.msu.edu/fact/hypoglycemia.html

UFO 58: SUBLUXATIONS

When misaligned vertebrae irritate or put pressure on spinal nerves, it is called a subluxation, a common condition that's often ignored. Symptoms include a stiff neck, headaches, and pain in the shoulders and back, as well as poor posture, anxiety, numbness, tingling, and frequent colds. Other symptoms are misaligned shoulders and hips and an arched lower back.

By adjusting, or realigning, the vertebrae that are out of place, a chiropractor can help relieve the pressure on spinal nerves. This adjustment can help ease symptoms right away or within a few days, but some people may require treatment for as long as several months.

Recommendations

1. See an experienced chiropractor or osteopath for help. X-rays can help to determine which vertebrae are misaligned.
2. Avoid high-impact activities that put stress on your spine and joints. Examples are running, basketball, plyometrics, and jumping rope (plyometrics are rapid movements that are performed with explosive force).

Books

The Chiropractor's Health Book: Simple, Natural Exercises for Relieving Headaches, Tension, and Back Pain by Leonard McGill. Crown, 1997.

Introduction to Chiropractic by Louis Sportelli. Practicemakers Products, 2000.

Chiropractic: Compassion and Expectation by Terry A. Rondberg and Timothy J. Feuling. SCB Distributors, 1999.

Web Links

www.chirolinks.com/chiropractic.htm
www.mtnchiro.com/conditions.htm
www.dcdoctor.com/pages/rightpages_allaboutchiro/subluxations.html

For a referral:

www.palmer.edu/pcc_alumni/dcreferrals.htm
www.amerchiro.org/aspdb/memsearch.asp

CHAPTER THREE

THE EXERCISE PROGRAM

If one knows and does not act, then one does not know.
                                                    UNKNOWN

The exercise plan in this chapter features techniques that are easy to learn. They're also some of the best I know for helping to save you time. The plan also features movements you can perform at a typical gym. If your gym doesn't have the machines you need, or you plan to work out at home, you can substitute some of the movements found at the end of Chapter Four. Whatever your fitness level is, this program should suit your needs as long as you make adjustments based on the way you respond and feel. For example, if you're on Cycle 3 and you find that it's too intense, instead of progressing to Cycle 4, repeat Cycle 3 the next week. But if Cycle 3 feels easy, skip right ahead to Cycle 4, or try moving slower, honing your form, and resting less time between sets.

Although the exercises you'll be performing are fairly routine, the way you're instructed to vary, combine, and execute them is unique. For example, you'll have to move at a speed that is much slower than the norm, and your rest intervals (between sets) will keep getting shorter as you progress. You'll also be training to "failure," which means until you are *fully* fatigued. Bear in mind, though, if you haven't trained much or you're currently not very fit, you may need a few weeks to work up to the point where failure can be achieved.

For a better idea of what's in store, consider the following points.

THE TEN MOST IMPORTANT COMPONENTS OF A SUCCESSFUL WEIGHT TRAINING ROUTINE

1. *It's simple.* If the program you follow is too complex or unnecessarily long, the odds that you will get bored and stop following it are extremely good. And the odds that you won't have any idea what you're doing are pretty good, too.

When your goal is to challenge your body, you should try not to challenge your mind. You'll find that it's hard enough to focus on one of these things at a time!

2. *It's short.* Contrary to what most people think or assume based on what they've heard, the best kind of workout is short and hard as opposed to long and lax. In fact, the harder (and better) you work, the shorter your workouts should be. You also should bear in mind that there is a point of diminishing gains; for example, training with weights for an hour or more can restrict your success. Rather than doing endless sets and hundreds of half-hearted reps, work harder, smarter, and slower and you'll discover that less is *more*.

3. *It's efficient.* For your workout to be efficient, making the most of your time is a must. This will require some vigilance on your part every time you train. You should also know that if you're inclined to spend too much time in the gym, it can lead to plateau phases, i.e., a failure to make further gains. There should be *no* wasted effort, extraneous movement, or needless rest! Not only must you not perform more sets than you truly need, you must also ensure that your rest intervals are not self-defeatingly long. Resting for more than one minute is, in most cases, ill advised unless you are training primarily to maximize gains in strength. Otherwise, to maximize gains in endurance, shape, and tone, your rest between sets should be minimal—meaning, don't waste a second of time!

4. *It's progressive.* To ensure that you keep making progress (and don't get frustrated or bored), it's important to change your routine over time in increasingly challenging ways. You can do this by resting less time between sets, slowing down, and honing your form, or changing your sequence of movements and exercise choices every few weeks. As you'll see, the following program gets more challenging every week. If you want to see your body and fitness level improve over time, you *must*, on a regular basis, vary some aspect of your routine.

5. *It's precise.* Too many people who exercise are careless and imprecise, ignoring critical factors that can make or break their success: for example, making adjustments based on their limb lengths, size, and shape, or changing their movement speed (or range) based on their limits and goals. It's important for you to be measured, detail oriented, and exact. Doing the little things right *all the time* is critical to your success—not only to prevent injury and ensure

that you keep making gains but also so the right muscle groups will always be properly stressed.

6. *It's focused.* The best type of workout is focused enough to put you into a "zone," one where you're mindful of each single movement you make and the way that it feels. It can even be meditative, if you approach it with that intent. Think of your workout as something that has the potential to mitigate stress or something that could be a whole new way of connecting your heart to your head. Use it to strengthen your body, of course, but also to strengthen your mind.

7. *It's safe.* If it puts too much stress on your body or has the potential to cause you harm, no program, no matter how "good" it is, is going to be worth your time. Too many people ignore the signs that their training techniques are unsafe and end up paying the price by injuring ligaments, muscles, and joints. Among the most common gaffes involving the use of machines and weights are being positioned improperly, arching the back, and moving too fast. Don't let yourself be a victim of limited knowledge or shoddy advice. Trust your body to tell you when you're putting yourself at risk.

8. *It's a challenge.* Here is what I've observed while working in gyms for the past twenty years: Nine out of every ten people don't work nearly as hard as they should. They basically go through the motions, ending each exercise on a whim, or they train for ridiculous lengths of time in a casual, effortless way. While I'm not of the mind that you need to get sick or pass out every time you train, I do feel a maximum effort is the key to a maximum gain. So really, instead of "no pain, no gain," it should be "no *effort*, no gain." Remember the following tip whenever you train with weights or machines: *Never* end any exercise after finishing one full rep; always make an effort to do a part of one rep more. This way, you'll know for sure that you've done as many reps as you can.

9. *It makes sense.* If you're like most people who exercise, i.e., "monkey see, monkey do," you probably really don't know for sure if what you've been doing makes sense. Here's what you need to be clear about before you trust any advice:

- It's based on reliable research and can be easily understood.
- It doesn't come from a trainer or coach with rigid or biased beliefs.
- It's right for you based on your body type, exercise history, health, and goals.

Beware of articulate "experts" who are devoid of common sense, for example, someone who eloquently suggests a one-week fast. Trust your intuition; always think before you act. Radical plans and rigid advice should always raise a red flag.

10. *It's flexible.* Here's why I feel the program in this book will fit the bill:

- It can be easily modified to meet individual needs; for example, you can repeat a week and proceed at a comfortable pace.
- It's based on exercises you can perform at any gym.

If a program is rigidly structured or designed for unusual needs, it's going to be hard to revise with regard to your personal goals and concerns. Ensure that the program you follow isn't too narrow or hard to adapt.

AEROBIC (CARDIOVASCULAR) EXERCISE

When performing aerobic exercise, consider the following points:

1. *Maintain your target heart rate (THR) when you work out.* You must maintain your THR to achieve your best result. If your heart rate exceeds your THR, your work load should be reduced. If it's lower than your THR, your work load should be increased. Use the following methods to determine your THR:

The Karvonen Formula
- Determine your resting heart rate (RHR) while lying in bed. With your fingers (not your thumb), locate your carotid or radial pulse. The carotid pulse can be found on either side of the front of your neck. The radial pulse can be found on the side of your wrist, below your thumb.
- 220 minus your age is your maximum heart rate (MHR).
- MHR minus RHR is your heart rate reserve (HRR).
- Multiply your HRR by 0.65 to 0.85 (0.65 if you're not in good shape, 0.85 if you are). The result will be your optimum target heart rate (THR).
- At five-minute intervals during your aerobic workout, check your pulse. Time yourself for six seconds while you count the number of beats. Add a zero to this number to determine your BPM (beats per minute). If you time yourself for ten seconds, multiply the result by six.

Modified Rating of Perceived Exertion (RPE)

- To assess your exertion accurately, experience is a must. You should have at least three weeks of aerobic training under your belt, otherwise you may misperceive your level of physical stress. Your level of intensity should generally be between 3 and 4 (3 if your fitness level is low and 4 if it is high).

Modified Rating Scale

1–A mild degree of effort with a minimal level of stress.
2–A mild to moderate effort with a low level of stress.
3–A moderate degree of effort (you can talk, but you'd rather not).
4–A high degree of effort (you can talk, but not for long).
5–A maximum level of effort (it's hard for you to speak).

Polar Heart Rate Monitor

- Visit the Polar website at www.polar.fi.

2. *In general, do* three *to* four *aerobic workouts every week.* It's best not to do more than four, but always try to do at least three.

3. *Plan to exercise one to three hours after you finish a meal.* If you exercise on a full stomach, it's likely to slow you down. If you train on an empty stomach, you're apt to feel sluggish, weak, and fatigued.

4. *Vary the time and intensity of your workouts during the week.*

5. *Incorporate interval training to provide a change of pace.* Rather than keep your intensity at the same level throughout your routine, go all out for thirty seconds, then go slow for the same length of time. You can also vary the intervals every week, if you prefer.

CARDIOVASCULAR FALLACIES
THAT CAN COMPROMISE YOUR SUCCESS

Fallacy #1: Train on an empty stomach—
first thing in the morning—to burn more fat.
This isn't false, per se, it's just that its value is overblown. For one thing, it's

hard to do and thus not worth the slight gain you *might* see. It's also a little risky to train when you've gone for so long without food (you'll feel weak and have little energy if your blood sugar level is low). You'll fare much better by training, instead, when you're at your physical peak.

Fallacy #2: Work out at a *lower* intensity to burn a *greater* amount of fat.

Again, this is misleading, although it does have a measure of truth. If your level of effort when training is low, you might burn a *little* more fat. However, if it is high, you'll actually burn more *after* the fact. So regardless of whether your workout is easy and long or hard and short, the amount of fat you'll lose in the end is likely to be the same.

Fallacy #3: To burn more fat, it's important to train for forty-five minutes or more.

The pros (the extra fat you might burn) are far outweighed by the cons. Training for forty-five minutes or more can overstress muscles and joints. It can also increase the time it takes to recover between routines.

Fallacy #4: To increase your aerobic fitness and the rate at which you burn fat, perform some type of aerobic routine at least *six* days a week.

In general, there's little advantage to training more than four times a week. Unless you're a world-class runner, Olympics contender, or Ironman champ, training more often than this can injure or weaken your muscles and joints. It may also increase your recovery time between sessions when training with weights.

RESISTANCE TRAINING

SET VARIATIONS

The following set variations will be the nucleus of your routine. For specific technique guidelines, refer to Chapter Four.

The Drop Set

- Start with the heaviest weight you can use to do six to twelve reps with strict form.

- When fully fatigued, lower the weight and *promptly* begin the next set.

The Delayed Drop Set

- Start with the heaviest weight you can use to do six to twelve reps with strict form.
- When fully fatigued, lower the weight and take a limited rest (bear in mind that your rest intervals should decrease as your fitness improves).

The Flush Set

- Perform two or more exercises in a row (for *one* muscle group)—for example, supine bench presses and flys—without any rest in between.

GENERAL GUIDELINES FOR CYCLES

- Don't proceed to the next cycle until you've mastered the one you're on. This means (a) you're not having trouble performing a certain technique, and (b) you've fully recovered before you begin your next routine.
- If you're just starting out or you don't have much experience lifting weights, begin with Cycle 1 and repeat until ready for Cycle 2.
- If you train with weights occasionally or have done so in the past, skip the first two cycles and begin with Cycle 3.
- If you're at a more advanced level, i.e., you've been lifting weights for years, skip the first five cycles and begin with Cycle 6.

SEQUENCING EXERCISE MODES

If you plan to perform an aerobic routine and train with weights on the same day, I strongly suggest you always do your weight training workout *first*. The reason for this is that when you lift weights in the manner advised in this book, your energy level must be high for your body to handle the stress. Because you're moving so slowly, training to failure, and taking short rests, fatiguing your muscles before you begin will prevent you from using good form.

Of course, you could always perform your aerobic routine on alternate days. If it's possible for you to do this, I recommend you give it a try, especially once your workouts start getting longer and more intense.

ISOLATION EXERCISES

To increase the size of your muscles and improve their shape and tone, I believe isolation movements are, in general, the way to go. I've never bought into the theory that to maximize muscular gains, muscles called "stabilizers" must be subjected to extra stress (stabilizers are muscle groups that help to support your joints). Strength coaches would take exception to this, as this theory is now in vogue, but to me the importance of training these muscle groups is overblown.

To understand my perspective, consider the use of exercise balls. Some experts think that by balancing on a ball while performing a lift, the aforementioned stabilizers will be stressed to a greater degree. Again, I don't buy the idea that this is a rational thing to do. Training correctly is hard enough without being perched on a ball! This will only cause injury (which I have witnessed *numerous* times). I've even seen people *stand* on a ball while performing presses and curls! This is what happens when people forget to filter advice through their brain (if you're thinking, "Hey, he's talking to *me*!," don't worry, you're not alone).

This doesn't mean that an exercise ball cannot be of any use. If it makes a movement more comfortable (and you can use it without falling off), this may be reason enough for you to include it in your routine. In fact, as long as you don't have to *work* to balance yourself on the ball, it can actually be a good way for you to vary the way you train: for example, by doing a squat with the ball between the wall and your back, or by resting your legs on the ball while doing a supine crunch.

RESISTANCE TRAINING CYCLES 1 AND 2

For Cycles 1 and 2: Perform this routine *three* days a week. Between each weight training session always take one full day of rest. Once you complete your third session, allow yourself *two* full days of rest. Never train the same muscle group (or groups) on consecutive days.

RESISTANCE TRAINING CYCLES 3 TO 12

For Cycles 3 to 12: Perform this routine *two* times a week. Between each weight training session always take two full days of rest. After the second session, you should always take three days of rest. Never train the same muscle group (or groups) on consecutive days.

Note: If you prefer, you may perform a *split* routine; for example, you may train different parts of your body on alternate days. If you do choose to split your workout, you should adhere to the following rule: Your upper back, biceps, triceps, and chest should always be trained on the same day. Beyond that, you may split your routine however you prefer, but don't deviate from the sequence recommended in this book.

Example of a Split Routine

Monday: upper body, cardio
Tuesday: lower body
Wednesday: cardio
Thursday: upper body, cardio
Friday: lower body
Saturday and Sunday: off

Please also note that when you're advised to take no rest between sets, this means you should change the resistance and proceed *without delay*. Make whatever adjustments you need to make as fast as you can, but don't rush so much that you risk getting hurt or using improper technique.

WARM-UP—ALL CYCLES

Perform a non–weight-bearing exercise at an easy or moderate pace (for example, cycling or walking at a slow, controlled rate of speed). On a scale of 1 to 5 (5 being as hard as you're able to work), strive to keep your intensity at a level of 2 or 3. Warm up for at least five minutes, but don't exceed fifteen.

POST-CYCLE STRETCH SEQUENCE

Repeat the stretches in sequence, always performing the quad stretch first. You can also repeat or add stretches depending on how different muscle groups feel.

REVISIONS TO CYCLES

As you move through the different cycles, various parts of your workout will change. These changes are in *italics* so they're easy to see at a glance.

REST INTERVALS

Don't begin timing your rest intervals until *you are ready to start*. You must be positioned correctly and your adjustments must all be secured.

- (0)   no rest between sets
- (30) 30-second rest
- (1)   1-minute rest

Record your rest intervals on your workout log (see pages 106–107). Mark the intervals next to the number of reps you do on the first set.

Example:

W	R
90 60	8 (0) 4
95 85	9 (30) 5

CYCLE I

RESISTANCE TRAINING

Quadriceps
Quad Stretch: 1 × each leg, 30-second (static) hold
Leg Extension: 1 set, 6–10 reps

Hamstrings
Hamstring Stretch: 1 × each leg, 30-second (static) hold
Seated Leg Curl: 1 set, 6–10 reps

Upper Back
Upper Back Stretch: 1 ×, 30-second (static) hold
Pulldown: 1 set, 6–10 reps

Biceps

Seated Biceps Curl (machine): 1 set, 6–10 reps

Calves

Calf Stretch: 1 × each side, 30-second (static) hold
Seated Calf Press (machine): 1 set, 8–12 reps

Chest

Chest Stretch: 1 ×, 30-second (static) hold
Vertical/Seated Chest Press (machine): 1 set, 6–10 reps

Triceps

Triceps Stretch: 1 × each arm, 30-second (static) hold
Triceps Extension (cable): 1 set, 6–10 reps

Abdominals

Supine Abdominal Crunch: 1 set, 8–12 reps

Shoulders

Shoulder Stretch: 1 ×, 30-second (static) hold
Seated Lateral Raise (dumbbell): 1 set, 6–10 reps

Lower Back

Lower Back Stretch: 1 ×, 30-second (static) hold
Lower Back Extension (machine): 1 set, 6–10 reps

CARDIOVASCULAR RX

Frequency: 3 days
Duration: 15–20 minutes (maintaining your THR)
Intensity: Determine your THR via the Karvonen formula (page 98).

CARDIOVASCULAR OPTIONS

Walking, elliptical cross-training, swimming, recumbent cycling, stationary cycling, low-impact aerobics, stepping, water aerobics, jogging. (If you've suffered a knee or back injury, high-impact movements are not advised.)

WORKOUT LOG

Name _____

Week _____

Exercise or Stretch	#	Seat Back	Seat Height	Leg Pad	Range Adj.	Technique Key	Date			
							Cycle			
							W	R	W	R

Technique Key

1. Never arch your lower back (make sure your spine is straight).
2. Try not to shrug your shoulders and/or tense your face and neck.
3. 1/2 range of motion.
4. 2/3 range of motion.
5. 3/4 range of motion.
6. Full range of motion.
7. Don't hold your breath (inhale as you lower, exhale as you lift).
8. Perform this movement SLOWLY (don't use momentum—maintain control).
9. Keep knees aligned with your feet (don't bow them in or out).
10. Keep your feet flat (don't raise your heels or push with the side of your foot).
11. Apply the force with your arms against the pads (don't use your hands).
12. Keep your feet together (or no more than an inch apart).
13. Position your feet (or hands) so they are 3" to 6" apart.

W	R	W	R	W	R	W	R	W	R	W	R	W	R

Technique Key, *continued*

14. Position feet (or hands) so they are 6" to 12" apart.
15. Position your feet (or hands) so they are 1' to 2' apart.
16. Keep your wrists as straight as you can and/or relax your grip.
17. Hold for one second once you have fully extended your arms or legs.
18. Hold for one second once you have fully flexed your arms or legs.
19. Maintain a *slight* arch in your lower back throughout the entire lift.
20. As you perform this exercise, do not pause at any point (keep continuous tension on the muscle you want to stress).
21. Always position your feet so they are pointed away from your shins.
22. Don't move your upper arms forward or your elbows away from your sides.
23. Stay in an upright position (never bend forward or lean back).
24. Keep your legs straight (if possible) or maintain a slight bend in your knees.

CYCLE 2

RESISTANCE TRAINING

Quadriceps

Quad Stretch: 1 × each leg, 30-second (static) hold

Leg Extension: 1st set, 6–10 reps *to failure; rest interval (1 minute); 2nd set, 4–8 reps to failure*

Hamstrings

Hamstring Stretch: 1 × each leg, 30-second (static) hold

Seated Leg Curl: 1 set, 6–10 reps *to failure*

Upper Back

Upper Back Stretch: 1 × each side, 30-second (static) hold

Pulldown: 1st set, 6–10 reps *to failure; rest interval (1 minute); 2nd set, 4–8 reps to failure*

Biceps

Seated Biceps Curl (machine): 1 set, 6–10 reps *to failure*

Calves

Calf Stretch: 1 × each side, 30-second (static) hold

Seated Calf Press (machine): 1 set, 8–12 reps *to failure*

Chest

Chest Stretch: 1 ×, 30-second (static) hold

Vertical/Seated Chest Press (machine): 1st set, 6–10 reps *to failure; rest interval (1 minute); 2nd set, 4–8 reps to failure*

Triceps

Triceps Stretch: 1 × each arm, 30-second (static) hold

Triceps Extension (cable): 1 set, 6–10 reps *to failure*

Abdominals

Supine Abdominal Crunch: 1st set, 8–12 reps *to failure; rest interval (1 minute); 2nd set, 6–10 reps to failure*

Shoulders
Shoulder Stretch: 1 ×, 30-second (static) hold
Seated Lateral Raise (dumbbell): 1 set, 6–10 reps *to failure*

Lower Back
Lower Back Stretch: 1 ×, 30-second (static) hold
Lower Back Extension (machine): 1 set, 6–10 reps *to failure*

CARDIOVASCULAR RX

Frequency: 3 days
Duration: *20 minutes (maintaining your THR)*
Intensity: Determine your THR via the Karvonen formula (page 98).

CARDIOVASCULAR OPTIONS

Walking, elliptical cross-training, swimming, recumbent cycling, stationary cycling, low-impact aerobics, stepping, water aerobics, jogging, *rowing*. (If you've suffered a knee or back injury, high-impact movements are not advised.)

CYCLE 3

RESISTANCE TRAINING

Quadriceps
Quad Stretch: 1 × each leg, 30-second (static) hold
Leg Extension: 1st set, 6–10 reps to failure; *rest interval (30 seconds);*
2nd set, 4–8 reps to failure

Hamstrings
Hamstring Stretch: 1 × each leg, 30-second (static) hold
Seated Leg Curl: 1st set, 6–10 reps to failure; *rest interval (1 minute);*
2nd set, 4–8 reps to failure

Upper Back

Upper Back Stretch: 1 ×, 30-second (static) hold

Pulldown: 1st set, 6–10 reps to failure; *rest interval (30 seconds);* 2nd set, 4–8 reps to failure

Biceps

Seated Biceps Curl (machine): 1st set, 6–10 reps to failure; *rest interval (1 minute); 2nd set, 4–8 reps to failure*

Calves

Calf Stretch: 1 × each side, 30-second (static) hold

Seated Calf Press (machine): 1st set, 8–12 reps to failure; *rest interval (1 minute); 2nd set, 6–10 reps to failure*

Chest

Chest Stretch: 1 ×, 30-second (static) hold

Vertical/Seated Chest Press (machine): 1st set, 6–10 reps to failure; *rest interval (30 seconds);* 2nd set, 4–8 reps to failure

Triceps

Triceps Stretch: 1 × each arm, 30-second (static) hold

Triceps Extension (cable): 1st set, 6–10 reps to failure; *rest interval (1 minute); 2nd set, 4–8 reps to failure*

Abdominals

Supine Abdominal Crunch: 1st set, 8–12 reps to failure; *rest interval (30 seconds);* 2nd set, 6–10 reps to failure

Shoulders

Shoulder Stretch: 1 ×, 30-second (static) hold

Seated Lateral Raise (dumbbell): 1st set, 6–10 reps to failure; *rest interval (1 minute); 2nd set, 4–8 reps to failure*

Lower Back

Lower Back Stretch: 1 ×, 30-second (static) hold

Lower Back Extension (machine): 1 set, 6–10 reps to failure

CARDIOVASCULAR RX

Frequency: 3 days
Duration: *2 days, 20 minutes at THR; 1 day, 25 minutes at THR*
Intensity: Determine your THR via the Karvonen formula (page 98).

CARDIOVASCULAR OPTIONS

Walking, elliptical cross-training, swimming, recumbent cycling, stationary cycling, low-impact aerobics, stepping, water aerobics, jogging, rowing, *Stair-Master*. (If you've suffered a knee or back injury, high-impact movements are not advised.)

CYCLE 4

RESISTANCE TRAINING

Quadriceps
Quad Stretch: 1 × each leg, 30-second (static) hold
Leg Extension: 1st set, 6–10 reps to failure; *rest interval (0 seconds);*
2nd set, 4–8 reps to failure
Leg Press (seated or supine): 1 set, 6–10 reps to failure

Hamstrings
Hamstring Stretch: 1 × each leg, 30-second (static) hold
Seated Leg Curl: 1st set, 6–10 reps to failure; *rest interval (30 seconds);*
2nd set, 4–8 reps to failure

Upper Back
Upper Back Stretch: 1 ×, 30-second (static) hold
Pulldown: 1st set, 6–10 reps to failure; *rest interval (0 seconds);* 2nd set,
4–8 reps to failure
Seated Row (cable): 1 set, 6–10 reps to failure

Biceps
Seated Biceps Curl (machine): 1st set, 6–10 reps to failure; *rest interval
(30 seconds);* 2nd set, 4–8 reps to failure

Calves

Calf Stretch: 1 × each side, 30-second (static) hold
Seated Calf Press (machine): 1st set, 8–12 reps to failure; *rest interval (30 seconds);* 2nd set, 6–10 reps to failure

Chest

Chest Stretch: 1 ×, 30-second (static) hold
Vertical/Seated Chest Press (machine): 1st set, 6–10 reps to failure; *rest interval (0 seconds);* 2nd set, 4–8 reps to failure
Pec Flys (machine): 1 set, 6–10 reps to failure

Triceps

Triceps Stretch: 1 × each arm, 30-second (static) hold
Triceps Extension (cable): 1st set, 6–10 reps to failure; *rest interval (30 seconds);* 2nd set, 4–8 reps to failure

Abdominals

Supine Abdominal Crunch: 1st set, 8–12 reps to failure; *rest interval (0 seconds);* 2nd set, 6–10 reps to failure

Shoulders

Shoulder Stretch: 1 ×, 30-second (static) hold
Seated Lateral Raise (dumbbell): 1st set, 6–10 reps to failure; *rest interval (30 seconds);* 2nd set, 4–8 reps to failure

Lower Back

Lower Back Stretch: 1 ×, 30-second (static) hold
Lower Back Extension (machine): 1 set, 6–10 reps to failure

CARDIOVASCULAR RX

Frequency: 3 days
Duration: *1 day, 20 minutes at THR; 2 days, 25 minutes at THR*
Intensity: Determine your THR via the Karvonen formula (page 98).

CARDIOVASCULAR OPTIONS

Walking, elliptical cross-training, swimming, recumbent cycling, stationary cycling, low-impact aerobics, stepping, water aerobics, jogging, rowing, Stair-Master, *spinning*. (If you've suffered a knee or back injury, high-impact movements are not advised.)

CYCLE 5

RESISTANCE TRAINING

Quadriceps
Quad Stretch: 1 × each leg, 30-second (static) hold
Leg Extension: 1st set, 6–10 reps to failure; rest interval (0 seconds);
2nd set, 4–8 reps to failure
Leg Press (seated or supine): 1st set, 6–10 reps to failure; *rest interval (1 minute); 2nd set, 4–8 reps to failure*

Hamstrings
Hamstring Stretch: 1 × each leg, 30-second (static) hold
Seated Leg Curl: 1st set, 6–10 reps to failure; *rest interval (0 seconds);* 2nd set, 4–8 reps to failure

Upper Back
Upper Back Stretch: 1 ×, 30-second (static) hold
Pulldown: 1st set, 6–10 reps to failure; rest interval (0 seconds); 2nd set, 4–8 reps to failure
Seated Row (cable): 1st set, 6–10 reps to failure; *rest interval (1 minute); 2nd set, 4–8 reps to failure*

Biceps
Seated Biceps Curl (machine): 1st set, 6–10 reps to failure; *rest interval (0 seconds);* 2nd set, 4–8 reps to failure

Calves
Calf Stretch: 1 × each side, 30-second (static) hold
Seated Calf Press (machine): 1st set, 8–12 reps to failure; *rest interval (0 seconds);* 2nd set, 6–10 reps to failure

Chest

Chest Stretch: 1 ×, 30-second (static) hold

Vertical/Seated Chest Press (machine): 1st set, 6–10 reps to failure; rest interval (0 seconds); 2nd set, 4–8 reps to failure

Pec Flys (machine): 1st set, 6–10 reps to failure; *rest interval (1 minute); 2nd set, 4–8 reps to failure*

Triceps

Triceps Stretch: 1 × each arm, 30-second (static) hold

Triceps Extension (cable): 1st set, 6–10 reps to failure; *rest interval (0 seconds); 2nd set, 4–8 reps to failure*

Triceps Extension (machine) or Triceps Press (machine): 1 set, 6–10 reps to failure

Abdominals

Supine Abdominal Crunch: 1st set, 8–12 reps to failure; rest interval (0 seconds); 2nd set, 6–10 reps to failure

Shoulders

Shoulder Stretch: 1 ×, 30-second (static) hold

Seated Lateral Raise (dumbbell): 1st set, 6–10 reps to failure; *rest interval (0 seconds); 2nd set, 4–8 reps to failure*

Seated Press (machine): 1 set, 6–10 reps to failure

Lower Back

Lower Back Stretch: 1 ×, 30-second (static) hold

Lower Back Extension (machine): 1 set, 6–10 reps to failure

CARDIOVASCULAR RX

Frequency: *3–4 days*

Duration: *2–3 days, 25 minutes at THR; 1 day, 30 minutes at THR*

Intensity: Determine your THR via the Karvonen formula (page 98).

CARDIOVASCULAR OPTIONS

Walking, elliptical cross-training, swimming, recumbent cycling, stationary cycling, low-impact aerobics, stepping, water aerobics, jogging, rowing, Stair-

Master, spinning, *powerwalking*. (If you've suffered a knee or back injury, high-impact movements are not advised.)

CYCLE 6

RESISTANCE TRAINING

Quadriceps
Quad Stretch: 1 × each leg, 30-second (static) hold
Leg Extension: 1st set, 6–10 reps to failure; rest interval (0 seconds); 2nd set, 4–8 reps to failure
Leg Press (seated or supine): 1st set, 6–10 reps to failure; *rest interval (30 seconds)*; 2nd set, 4–8 reps to failure

Hamstrings
Hamstring Stretch: 1 × each leg, 30-second (static) hold
Seated Leg Curl: 1st set, 6–10 reps to failure; rest interval (0 seconds); 2nd set, 4–8 reps to failure

Upper Back
Upper Back Stretch: 1 ×, 30-second (static) hold
Pulldown: 1st set, 6–10 reps to failure; rest interval (0 seconds); 2nd set, 4–8 reps to failure
Seated Row (cable): 1st set, 6–10 reps to failure; *rest interval (30 seconds)*; 2nd set, 4–8 reps to failure

Biceps
Seated Biceps Curl (machine): 1st set, 6–10 reps to failure; rest interval (0 seconds); 2nd set, 4–8 reps to failure
Standing Biceps Curl (cable): 1 set, 6–10 reps to failure

Calves
Calf Stretch: 1 × each side, 30-second (static) hold
Seated Calf Press (machine): 1st set, 8–12 reps to failure; rest interval (0 seconds); 2nd set, 6–10 reps to failure

Chest
Chest Stretch: 1 ×, 30-second (static) hold
Vertical/Seated Chest Press (machine): 1st set, 6–10 reps to failure; rest

interval (0 seconds); 2nd set, 4–8 reps to failure

Pec Flys (machine): 1st set, 6–10 reps to failure; *rest interval (30 seconds);* 2nd set, 4–8 reps to failure

Triceps

Triceps Stretch: 1 × each arm, 30-second (static) hold

Triceps Extension (cable): 1st set, 6–10 reps to failure; rest interval (0 seconds); 2nd set, 4–8 reps to failure

Triceps Extension (machine) or Triceps Press (machine): 1st set, 6–10 reps to failure; *rest interval (1 minute); 2nd set, 4–8 reps to failure*

Abdominals

Abdominal Crunch (machine): 1 set, 8–12 reps to failure

Supine Abdominal Crunch: 1st set, 8–12 reps to failure; rest interval (0 seconds); 2nd set, 6–10 reps to failure

Shoulders

Shoulder Stretch: 1 ×, 30-second (static) hold

Seated Lateral Raise (dumbbell): 1st set, 6–10 reps to failure; rest interval (0 seconds); 2nd set, 4–8 reps to failure

Seated Press (machine): 1st set, 6–10 reps to failure; *rest interval (1 minute); 2nd set, 4–8 reps to failure*

Lower Back

Lower Back Stretch: 1 ×, 30-second (static) hold

Lower Back Extension (machine): 1 set, 6–10 reps to failure

CARDIOVASCULAR RX

Frequency: 3–4 days

Duration: *2 days, 25 minutes at THR; 1–2 days, 30 minutes at THR*

Intensity: Determine your THR via the Karvonen formula (page 98) *or by using the Modified Rating of Perceived Exertion scale* (page 99).

CARDIOVASCULAR OPTIONS

Walking, elliptical cross-training, swimming, recumbent cycling, stationary cycling, low-impact aerobics, stepping, water aerobics, jogging, rowing, Stair-

Master, spinning, powerwalking, *interval training* (see explanation on page 99). (If you've suffered a knee or back injury, high-impact movements are not advised.)

CYCLE 7

RESISTANCE TRAINING

Quadriceps

Quad Stretch: 1 × each leg, 30-second (static) hold
Leg Extension: 1st set, 6–10 reps to failure; rest interval (0 seconds); 2nd set, 4–8 reps to failure
Leg Press (seated or supine): 1st set, 6–10 reps to failure; *rest interval (0 seconds);* 2nd set, 4–8 reps to failure

Hamstrings

Hamstring Stretch: 1 × each leg, 30-second (static) hold
Seated Leg Curl: 1st set, 6–10 reps to failure; rest interval (0 seconds); 2nd set, 4–8 reps to failure

Upper Back

Upper Back Stretch: 1 ×, 30-second (static) hold
Pulldown: 1st set, 6–10 reps to failure; rest interval (0 seconds); 2nd set, 4–8 reps to failure
Seated Row (cable): 1st set, 6–10 reps to failure; *rest interval (0 seconds);* 2nd set, 4–8 reps to failure

Biceps

Seated Biceps Curl (machine): 1st set, 6–10 reps to failure; rest interval (0 seconds); 2nd set, 4–8 reps to failure
Standing Biceps Curl (cable): 1st set, 6–10 reps to failure; *rest interval (1 minute); 2nd set, 4–8 reps to failure*

Calves

Calf Stretch: 1 × each side, 30-second (static) hold
Standing Calf Raise (machine): 1 set, 8–12 reps to failure
Seated Calf Press (machine): 1st set, 8–12 reps to failure; rest interval (0 seconds); 2nd set, 6–10 reps to failure

Chest

Chest Stretch: 1 ×, 30-second (static) hold
Vertical/Seated Chest Press (machine): 1st set, 6–10 reps to failure; rest interval (0 seconds); 2nd set, 4–8 reps to failure
Pec Flys (machine): 1st set, 6–10 reps to failure; *rest interval (0 seconds)*; 2nd set, 4–8 reps to failure

Triceps

Triceps Stretch: 1 × each arm, 30-second (static) hold
Triceps Extension (cable): 1st set, 6–10 reps to failure; rest interval (0 seconds); 2nd set, 4–8 reps to failure
Triceps Extension (machine) or Triceps Press (machine): 1st set, 6–10 reps to failure; *rest interval (30 seconds)*; 2nd set, 4–8 reps to failure

Abdominals

Abdominal Crunch (machine): 1st set, 8–12 reps to failure; *rest interval (1 minute); 2nd set, 6–10 reps to failure*
Supine Abdominal Crunch: 1st set, 8–12 reps to failure; rest interval (0 seconds); 2nd set, 6–10 reps to failure

Shoulders

Shoulder Stretch: 1 ×, 30-second (static) hold
Seated Lateral Raise (dumbbell): 1st set, 6–10 reps to failure; rest interval (0 seconds); 2nd set, 4–8 reps to failure
Seated Press (machine): 1st set, 6–10 reps to failure; *rest interval (30 seconds)*; 2nd set, 4–8 reps to failure

Lower Back

Lower Back Stretch: 1 ×, 30-second (static) hold
Lower Back Extension (machine): 1st set, 6–10 reps to failure; *rest interval (1 minute); 2nd set, 4–8 reps to failure*

CARDIOVASCULAR RX

Frequency: 3–4 days
Duration: *1 day, 25 minutes at THR; 2–3 days, 30 minutes at THR*
Intensity: Determine your THR via the Karvonen formula (page 98) or by using the Modified Rating of Perceived Exertion Scale (page 99).

CARDIOVASCULAR OPTIONS

Walking, elliptical cross-training, swimming, recumbent cycling, stationary cycling, low-impact aerobics, stepping, water aerobics, jogging, rowing, Stair-Master, spinning, powerwalking, interval training, *step aerobics*. (If you've suffered a knee or back injury, high-impact movements are not advised.)

CYCLE 8

Perform all bracketed movements in succession without any rest. Adjust the position of pads, resistance, and seat without delay.

RESISTANCE TRAINING

Quadriceps

Quad Stretch: 1 × each leg, 30-second (static) hold
[Leg Press (seated or supine): 1st set, 6–10 reps to failure; rest interval (0 seconds); 2nd set, 4–8 reps to failure]
[Leg Extension: *1 set*, 6–10 reps to failure]

Hamstrings

Hamstring Stretch: 1 × each leg, 30-second (static) hold
Prone Leg Curl: 1 set, 6–10 reps to failure
Seated Leg Curl: *1 set*, 6–10 reps to failure

Upper Back

Upper Back Stretch: 1 ×, 30-second (static) hold
[Seated Row (cable): 1st set, 6–10 reps to failure; rest interval (0 seconds); 2nd set, 4–8 reps to failure]
[Pulldown: *1 set*, 6–10 reps to failure]

Biceps

Seated Dumbbell Curl: 1 set, 6–10 reps to failure
Standing Biceps Curl (cable): 1st set, 6–10 reps to failure; *rest interval (30 seconds)*; 2nd set, 4–8 reps to failure

Calves

Calf Stretch: 1 × each side, 30-second (static) hold

Standing Calf Raise (machine): 1st set, 8–12 reps to failure; *rest interval (1 minute); 2nd set, 6–10 reps to failure*

Seated Calf Press (machine): 1st set, 8–12 reps to failure; rest interval (0 seconds); 2nd set, 6–10 reps to failure

Chest

Chest Stretch: 1 ×, 30-second (static) hold

Free Weight Bench Press (supine): 1 warm-up set (50% of your 1-rep max); 1 set, 6–10 reps to failure

Pec Flys (machine): 1st set, 6–10 reps to failure; rest interval (0 seconds); 2nd set, 4–8 reps to failure

Triceps

Triceps Stretch: 1 × each arm, 30-second (static) hold

Triceps Extension (dumbbell): 1 set, 6–10 reps to failure

Triceps Extension (machine) or Triceps Press (machine): 1st set, 6–10 reps to failure; *rest interval (0 seconds);* 2nd set, 4–8 reps to failure

Abdominals

Abdominal Crunch (machine): 1 set, 8–12 reps to failure; *rest interval (30 seconds);* 2nd set, 6–10 reps to failure

Supine Abdominal Crunch: 1st set, 8–12 reps to failure; rest interval (0 seconds); 2nd set, 6–10 reps to failure

Shoulders

Shoulder Stretch: 1 ×, 30-second (static) hold

Seated Lateral Raise (machine): 1 set, 6–10 reps to failure

Seated Press (machine): 1st set, 6–10 reps to failure; *rest interval (0 seconds);* 2nd set, 4–8 reps to failure

Lower Back

Lower Back Stretch: 1 ×, 30-second (static) hold

Lower Back Extension (machine): 1st set, 6–10 reps to failure; *rest interval (30 seconds);* 2nd set, 4–8 reps to failure

CARDIOVASCULAR RX

Frequency: 3–4 days
Duration: *3–4 days, 30 minutes at THR*
Intensity: Determine your THR via the Karvonen formula (page 98) or by using the Modified Rating of Perceived Exertion scale (page 99).

CARDIOVASCULAR OPTIONS

Walking, elliptical cross-training, swimming, recumbent cycling, stationary cycling, low-impact aerobics, stepping, water aerobics, jogging, rowing, Stair-Master, spinning, powerwalking, interval training, step aerobics, *jazz, funk, or dance aerobics.* (If you've suffered a knee or back injury, high-impact movements are not advised.)

CYCLE 9

Perform all bracketed movements in succession without any rest. Adjust the position of pads, resistance, and seat without delay.

RESISTANCE TRAINING

Quadriceps
Quad Stretch: 1 × each leg, 30-second (static) hold
[Leg Press (seated or supine): *1 set, 6–10 reps to failure*]
[Leg Extension: 1st set, 6–10 reps to failure; *rest interval (0 seconds);*
2nd set, 4–8 reps to failure]

Hamstrings
Hamstring Stretch: 1 × each leg, 30-second (static) hold
Prone Leg Curl: 1st set, 6–10 reps to failure; *rest interval (1 minute);*
2nd set, 4–8 reps to failure

Upper Back

Upper Back Stretch: 1 ×, 30-second (static) hold

[Seated Row (cable): *1 set, 6–10 reps to failure*]

[Pulldown: 1st set, 6–10 reps to failure; *rest interval (0 seconds); 2nd set, 4–8 reps to failure*]

Biceps

Seated Dumbbell Curl: 1st set, 6–10 reps to failure; *rest interval (1 minute); 2nd set, 4–8 reps to failure*

Standing Biceps Curl (cable): 1st set, 6–10 reps to failure; *rest interval (0 seconds);* 2nd set, 4–8 reps to failure

Calves

Calf Stretch: 1 × each side, 30-second (static) hold

Standing Calf Raise (machine): 1st set, 8–12 reps to failure; *rest interval (30 seconds);* 2nd set, 6–10 reps to failure

Seated Calf Press (machine): 1st set, 8–12 reps to failure; rest interval (0 seconds); 2nd set, 6–10 reps to failure

Chest

Chest Stretch: 1 ×, 30-second (static) hold

[Free Weight Bench Press (supine): 1 warm-up set (50% of your 1-rep max); 1st set, 6–10 reps to failure; *rest interval (1 minute); 2nd set, 4–8 reps to failure*]

[Pec Flys (machine): *1 set,* 6–10 reps to failure]

Triceps

Triceps Stretch: 1 × each arm, 30-second (static) hold

[Triceps Extension (dumbbell): 1st set, 6–10 reps to failure; *rest interval (1 minute); 2nd set, 4–8 reps to failure*]

[Triceps Extension (machine) or Triceps Press (machine): *1 set,* 6–10 reps to failure]

Abdominals

Abdominal Crunch (machine): 1st set, 8–12 reps to failure; *rest interval (0 seconds);* 2nd set, 6–10 reps to failure

Supine Abdominal Crunch: 1st set, 8–12 reps to failure; rest interval (0 seconds); 2nd set, 6–10 reps to failure

Shoulders

Shoulder Stretch: 1 ×, 30-second (static) hold

[Seated Lateral Raise (machine): 1st set, 6–10 reps to failure; *rest interval (1 minute); 2nd set, 4–8 reps to failure*]

[Seated Press (machine): *1 set*, 6–10 reps to failure]

Lower Back

Lower Back Stretch: 1 ×, 30-second (static) hold

Lower Back Extension (machine): 1st set, 6–10 reps to failure; *rest interval (0 seconds)*; 2nd set, 4–8 reps to failure

CARDIOVASCULAR RX

Frequency: *4 days*

Duration: *3 days, 30 minutes at THR; 1 day, 35 minutes at THR*

Intensity: Determine your THR via the Karvonen formula (page 98) or by using the Modified Rating of Perceived Exertion scale (page 99).

CARDIOVASCULAR OPTIONS

Walking, elliptical cross-training, swimming, recumbent cycling, stationary cycling, low-impact aerobics, stepping, water aerobics, jogging, rowing, Stair-Master, spinning, powerwalking, interval training, step aerobics, jazz, funk, or dance aerobics, *running (low to moderate intensity)*. (If you've suffered a knee or back injury, high impact movements are not advised.)

CYCLE 10

Perform all bracketed movements in succession without any rest. Adjust the position of pads, resistance, and seat without delay.

RESISTANCE TRAINING

Quadriceps

Quad Stretch: 1 × each leg, 30-second (static) hold

[Leg Extension: *1 set, 6–10 reps to failure*]
[Leg Press (seated or supine): 1 set, 6–10 reps to failure; *rest interval (0 seconds); 2nd set, 4–8 reps to failure*]

Hamstrings

Hamstring Stretch: 1 × each leg, 30-second (static) hold
Prone Leg Curl: 1st set, 6–10 reps to failure; *rest interval (30 seconds);* 2nd set, 4–8 reps to failure

Upper Back

Upper Back Stretch: 1 ×, 30-second (static) hold
[Pulldown: *1 set, 6–10 reps to failure*]
[Seated Row (cable): 1st set, 6–10 reps to failure; *rest interval (0 seconds); 2nd set, 4–8 reps to failure*]

Biceps

Seated Dumbbell Curl: 1st set, 6–10 reps to failure; *rest interval (30 seconds);* 2nd set, 4–8 reps to failure
Seated Hammer Curl (dumbbell): 1 set, 6–10 reps to failure

Calves

Calf Stretch: 1 × each side, 30-second (static) hold
[Standing Calf Raise (machine): 1st set, 8–12 reps to failure; *rest interval (0 seconds);* 2nd set, 6–10 reps to failure]
[Seated Calf Press (machine): *1 set,* 8–12 reps to failure]

Chest

Chest Stretch: 1 ×, 30-second (static) hold
[Free Weight Bench Press (supine): 1 warm-up set (50% of your 1-rep max); 1st set, 6–10 reps to failure; *rest interval (30 seconds);* 2nd set, 4–8 reps to failure]
[Pec Flys (machine): 1 set, 6–10 reps to failure]

Triceps

Triceps Stretch: 1 × each arm, 30-second (static) hold
[Triceps Extension (dumbbell): 1st set, 6–10 reps to failure; *rest interval (30 seconds);* 2nd set, 4–8 reps to failure]
[Triceps Extension (machine) or Triceps Press (machine): 1 set, 6–10 reps to failure]

Abdominals

Abdominal Crunch (supine/alternate twist): 1 set, 8–12 reps to failure
Abdominal Crunch (machine): 1st set, 8–12 reps to failure; rest interval
(0 seconds); 2nd set, 6–10 reps to failure

Shoulders

Shoulder Stretch: 1 ×, 30-second (static) hold
[Seated Lateral Raise (machine): 1 set, 6–10 reps to failure; *rest interval
(30 seconds)*; 2nd set, 4–8 reps to failure]
[Seated Press (machine): 1 set, 6–10 reps to failure]

Lower Back

Lower Back Stretch: 1 ×, 30-second (static) hold
Lower Back Extension (machine): 1 set, 6–10 reps to failure; rest interval
(0 seconds); 2nd set, 4–8 reps to failure

CARDIOVASCULAR RX

Frequency: 4 days
Duration: *2 days, 30 minutes at THR; 2 days, 35 minutes at THR*
Intensity: Determine your THR via the Karvonen formula (page 98) or
by using the Modified Rating of Perceived Exertion scale (page 99).

CARDIOVASCULAR OPTIONS

Walking, elliptical cross-training, swimming, recumbent cycling, stationary
cycling, low-impact aerobics, stepping, water aerobics, jogging, rowing, Stair-
Master, spinning, powerwalking, interval training, step aerobics, jazz, funk,
or dance aerobics, running (low to moderate intensity), *rockclimbing (rock
wall)*. (If you've suffered a knee or back injury, high-impact movements are
not advised.)

CYCLE 11

Perform all bracketed movements in succession without any rest. Adjust the
position of pads, resistance, and seat without delay.

RESISTANCE TRAINING

Quadriceps

Quad Stretch: 1 × each leg, 30-second (static) hold

[Leg Extension: 1st set, 6–10 reps to failure; *rest interval (0 seconds);* *2nd set, 4–8 reps to failure*]

[Leg Press (seated or supine): *1 set,* 6–10 reps to failure]

45-Degree Hack Squat (machine): 1 set, 6–10 reps to failure

Hamstrings

Hamstring Stretch: 1 × each leg, 30-second (static) hold

Prone Leg Curl: 1st set, 6–10 reps to failure; *rest interval (0 seconds);* 2nd set, 4–8 reps to failure

Upper Back

Upper Back Stretch: 1 ×, 30-second (static) hold

[Pulldown: 1st set, 6–10 reps to failure; *rest interval (0 seconds); 2nd set, 4–8 reps to failure*]

[Seated Row (cable): *1 set,* 6–10 reps to failure]

Biceps

Seated Dumbbell Curl: 1st set, 6–10 reps to failure; *rest interval (0 seconds);* 2nd set, 4–8 reps to failure

Seated Hammer Curl (dumbbell): 1st set, 6–10 reps to failure; *rest interval (1 minute); 2nd set, 4–8 reps to failure*

Calves

Calf Stretch: 1 × each side, 30-second (static) hold

[Seated Calf Press (machine): 1st set, 8–12 reps to failure; *rest interval (0 seconds); 2nd set, 6–10 reps to failure*]

[Standing Calf Raise (machine): *1 set,* 8–12 reps to failure]

Chest

Chest Stretch: 1 ×, 30-second (static) hold

[Free Weight Bench Press (supine): 1 warm-up set (50% of your 1-rep max); 1st set, 6–10 reps to failure; *rest interval (0 seconds);* 2nd set, 4–8 reps to failure]

[Pec Flys (machine): 1st set, 6–10 reps to failure; *rest interval (1 minute); 2nd set, 4–8 reps to failure*]

Triceps

Triceps Stretch: 1 × each arm, 30-second (static) hold
[Triceps Extension (dumbbell): 1st set, 6–10 reps to failure; *rest interval (0 seconds)*; 2nd set, 4–8 reps to failure]
[Triceps Extension (machine) or Triceps Press (machine): 1 set, 6–10 reps to failure]

Abdominals

Abdominal Crunch (supine/alternate twist): 1st set, 8–12 reps to failure; *rest interval (1 minute); 2nd set, 6–10 reps to failure*
Abdominal Crunch (machine): 1st set, 8–12 reps to failure; rest interval (0 seconds); 2nd set, 6–10 reps to failure

Shoulders

Shoulder Stretch: 1 ×, 30-second (static) hold
[Seated Lateral Raise (machine): 1st set, 6–10 reps to failure; *rest interval (0 seconds)*; 2nd set, 4–8 reps to failure]
[Seated Press (machine): 1 set, 6–10 reps to failure]

Lower Back

Lower Back Stretch: 1 ×, 30-second (static) hold
Lower Back Extension (machine): 1st set, 6–10 reps to failure; rest interval (0 seconds); 2nd set, 4–8 reps to failure

CARDIOVASCULAR RX

Frequency: 4 days
Duration: *1 day, 30 minutes at THR; 3 days, 35 minutes at THR*
Intensity: Determine your THR via the Karvonen formula (page 98) or by using the Modified Rating of Perceived Exertion scale (page 99).

CARDIOVASCULAR OPTIONS

Walking, elliptical cross-training, swimming, recumbent cycling, stationary cycling, low-impact aerobics, stepping, water aerobics, jogging, rowing, Stair-Master, spinning, powerwalking, interval training, step aerobics, jazz, funk, or dance aerobics, running (low to moderate intensity), rockclimbing (rock wall), *boxing (speed or heavy bag)*. (If you've suffered a knee or back injury, high-impact movements are not advised.)

CYCLE 12

Perform all bracketed movements in succession without any rest. Adjust the position of pads, resistance, and seat without delay.

RESISTANCE TRAINING

Quadriceps

Quad Stretch: 1 × each leg, 30-second (static) hold
Leg Extension: 1st set, 6–10 reps to failure; rest interval (0 seconds); 2nd set, 4–8 reps to failure
[Leg Press (seated or supine): 1 set, 6–10 reps to failure]
[45-Degree Hack Squat (machine): 1 set, 6–10 reps to failure]

Hamstrings

Hamstring Stretch: 1 × each leg, 30-second (static) hold
[Prone Leg Curl: *1 set,* 6–10 reps to failure]
[*Seated Leg Curl: 1 set, 6–10 reps to failure*]

Upper Back

Upper Back Stretch: 1 ×, 30-second (static) hold
[Seated Row (cable): 1 set, 6–10 reps to failure; *rest interval (0 seconds); 2nd set, 4–8 reps to failure*]
[Pulldown: *1 set,* 6–10 reps to failure]

Biceps

[Seated Dumbbell Curl: 1 set, 6–10 reps to failure; rest interval (0 seconds); 2nd set, 4–8 reps to failure]
[Seated Hammer Curl (dumbbell): 1st set, 6–10 reps to failure; *rest interval (30 seconds)*; 2nd set, 4–8 reps to failure]

Calves

Calf Stretch: 1 × each side, 30-second (static) hold
[Standing Calf Raise (machine): 1st set, 8–12 reps to failure; *rest interval*

(0 seconds); *2nd set, 6–10 reps to failure*]
[Seated Calf Press (machine): *1 set,* 8–12 reps to failure]

Chest

Chest Stretch: 1 ×, 30-second (static) hold
[Free Weight Bench Press (supine): 1 warm-up set (50% of your 1-rep max); 1st set, 6–10 reps to failure; rest interval (0 seconds); 2nd set, 4–8 reps to failure]
[Pec Flys (machine): 1st set, 6–10 reps to failure; *rest interval (30 seconds);* 2nd set, 4–8 reps to failure]

Triceps

Triceps Stretch: 1 × each arm, 30-second (static) hold
[Triceps Extension (machine) or Triceps Press (machine): 1st set, 6–10 reps to failure; *rest interval (0 seconds); 2nd set, 4–8 reps to failure*]
[Triceps Extension (dumbbell): *1 set,* 6–10 reps to failure]

Abdominals

[Abdominal Crunch (supine/alternate twist): 1st set, 8–12 reps to failure; *rest interval (30 seconds);* 2nd set, 6–10 reps to failure]
[Abdominal Crunch (machine): *1 set,* 8–12 reps to failure]

Shoulders

Shoulder Stretch: 1 ×, 30-second (static) hold
[Seated Press (machine): 1st set, 6–10 reps to failure; *rest interval (0 seconds); 2nd set, 4–8 reps to failure*]
[Seated Lateral Raise (machine): *1 set,* 6–10 reps to failure]

Lower Back

Lower Back Stretch: 1 ×, 30-second (static) hold
Lower Back Extension (machine): 1st set, 6–10 reps to failure; rest interval (0 seconds); 2nd set, 4–8 reps to failure

CARDIOVASCULAR RX

Frequency: 4 days
Duration: *4 days, 35 minutes at THR*

Intensity: Determine your THR via the Karvonen formula (page 98) or by using the Modified Rating of Perceived Exertion scale (page 99).

CARDIOVASCULAR OPTIONS

Walking, elliptical cross-training, swimming, recumbent cycling, stationary cycling, low-impact aerobics, stepping, water aerobics, jogging, rowing, Stair-Master, spinning, powerwalking, interval training, step aerobics, jazz, funk, or dance aerobics, running (low to moderate intensity), rockclimbing (rock wall), boxing (speed or heavy bag). (If you've suffered a knee or back injury, high-impact movements are not advised.)

CHAPTER FOUR

THE RESISTANCE EXERCISES

If fifty million people say a foolish thing, it is still a foolish thing.
                                                        ANATOLE FRANCE

I'll never forget the day a friend called, upset about something he'd read. "Did you see the *Newsweek* piece?" he asked. "Somebody ripped off your idea! It's all about how training slowly with weights provides faster and better results! Weren't you the one who discovered this first? Why didn't they interview you? Why don't you write to the magazine and tell them who you are!"

Now although I was touched and amused that he was so miffed on my behalf, the truth is that this is *not* my idea and it's not even all that new (the inventor of Nautilus, Arthur Jones, was the first to profess its worth). But in spite of the "newfound" research touting the value of slow exercise, proponents of slow-movement training are, and may always be, on the fringe. The reasons for this run the gamut, from people who worry about looking strange to others who balk at any idea that necessitates using less weight. I've also heard people express concern that their workouts will take too long (in fact, they'd have to do fewer sets, meaning much *less* time in the gym!). And, of course, there are those who are still unaware that this "new" approach even exists.

SLOW-MO IS THE WAY TO GO

Pure and simple, here's the scoop about working out slowly with weights: If you train this way, you'll avoid getting hurt and get markedly better results. This is because the faster you move, the more different muscles you use, which means that the muscle you're targeting does not get sufficiently stressed. To illustrate, if you move quickly when performing a biceps curl, you're likely to shrug your shoulders, bend your legs, and arch your back. And the more you do, the less involved your biceps will be in the lift. Conversely, when you move slowly, the muscles you're targeting do more work. Not only that, but you're less apt to suffer from tears and overstressed joints.

You may also find that working out slowly has meditative effects. Because you'll be much more focused, you'll be more conscious of how you feel. And paying attention to how you feel is going to improve your result.

Slow-movement training takes discipline, but believe me, the payoff is great. With well over twenty years of studying, teaching, and using this technique, I have all the proof I need that training this way leads to greater gains. In fact, it makes such a difference that it is often beyond belief.

Consider the following guidelines when you perform your weight training routine:

- In order to train more slowly, you will have to use less weight. Start by using 60 percent of the weight you normally use. Remember, it's not how *much* you use, it's *how* you use it that counts!
- While the lifting phase of most movements should be four to six seconds long, the duration of the lowering phase should be about six to eight (this will vary depending on how far you have to move). Presumably, this is *much* slower than you usually move when you train. Expect this to feel a bit awkward at first, as well as a lot more intense. With practice and patience, however, you'll adjust to the rhythm and flow, and once you do, you'll come to appreciate why this approach is advised.
- If you can't do at least six reps, reduce the weight next time you work out. If you're able to do ten reps with perfect form, increase the weight. (Please note that for some exercises, the optimum range is eight to twelve.)

TRAINING TO MUSCULAR FAILURE

Training to muscular failure will maximize gains in strength and tone unless you're just starting to exercise or the following errors are made:

- A muscle group is maximally stressed more than twice a week.
- You train the same muscle group (maximally) two or more days in a row.

- You perform more sets than you need to, or an exercise is performed wrong.
- You're ill, have an injury, haven't warmed up, or try to lift too much weight.

GUIDELINES FOR TRAINING TO FAILURE

1. *Never end an exercise after completing one full rep.* Always make an effort to do at least a little bit more; for example, do one-fourth, one-half, or three-fourths of another full rep.

2. *Anticipate how many reps you can do (for example, imagine it's ten).* Then choose a higher number (twelve) and count your reps *backward* (to one). Doing this can be disorienting—but in a productive way. You'll forget about how many reps you've done and how many more you "should" do.

3. *Enlist a spotter to motivate you to do those last few reps.* Could it be that you're limited less by your body than you are by your mind? I often "trick" people to do more reps than they really believe they can. When I place my hand below the bar and they think I'm assisting their lift, almost without exception they find a sudden reserve of strength!

SEQUENCE OF EXERCISES

Here is the rationale for the sequence of movements you'll perform:

- Perform all your upper-thigh movements first, while your energy is at its peak.
- Because you need maximum gripping strength to perform pulldowns and rows, train your upper back next, before your hands, wrists, and forearms fatigue.
- Always train your biceps after you've trained your upper back. Because your biceps are heavily stressed when you perform pulldowns and rows, this muscle group won't need a warm-up and will already be prestretched.
- Train your calves after your biceps to give your shoulders and arms a rest.
- If possible, train your chest and triceps after you've trained your calves. So your triceps won't fatigue before your chest is maximally

stressed, always work your triceps immediately after you've trained your chest.

- After your triceps, train your abs (to rest your shoulders and arms).
- To prevent your shoulders from tiring before other muscles are maximally stressed, always train them after you've trained your arms, upper back, and chest.
- Always do lower-back movements at the *end* of your routine. If you tire your lower back muscles before you train other muscle groups, you'll find yourself feeling unstable, using poor form, and arching your back. Your back must be strong to support your spine throughout your entire routine.
- Inner and outer thigh movements aren't included in this routine, as the muscles that these movements target rarely require any extra work. Since the problem that most people have is excess fat as opposed to poor tone, focusing on the hips and inner thighs is not advised. Remember, there are no movements that will help you spot reduce!

THE RESISTANCE EXERCISES

Whenever I read a description of how an exercise should be performed, I question why so many basic details are missing or poorly explained. More often than not, the instructions are either all wrong or laughably vague. For example, "Sit down, lift weight, get off" is not really very much help. Okay, so maybe it's not *that* bad, but I'm trying to make a point. And the point is that I think you need more help than you usually get.

With this in mind, consider the following ways to perfect your technique. Remember, addressing these details will do much to improve your results. Be sure to review them frequently to gradually hone your form.

QUADRICEPS

Leg Extension (Machine)

1. Select a weight that you're able to use for six to ten reps with strict form.
2. Adjust the leg pad to accommodate the length of your lower leg (the pad should rest on the curve between your shin and the top of your foot).

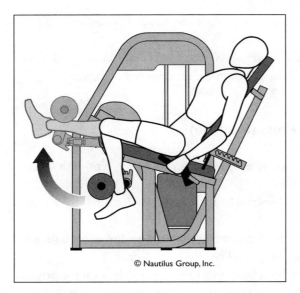

© Nautilus Group, Inc.

Figure 4.1
Leg Extension

3. Once you are seated on the machine, move the seat forward or back (the lowermost part of the seat back should be an inch from your lower back).
4. Ensure that your "pivotal joint" is aligned with the centerpoint of the cam (when performing the leg extension, the pivotal joint is your knee).
5. Position your lower legs behind the leg, or "roller," pads.
6. Fasten the seat belt snugly, so that you can't lift your hips from the seat.
7. Ensure that your knees and feet are roughly 4 to 10 inches apart.
8. Lean back on the seat and place your hands very lightly on the grips.
9. Extend your legs very slowly, pointing your feet *away* from your shins.
10. Pause for one full second once you've fully extended your legs.
11. Lower the weight very slowly, keeping your movement under control.
12. Stop just before the point at which your thighs are minimally stressed (1 to 2 inches above the point where the plates would touch the stack).
13. Repeat until you reach failure (you can't perform any more reps with strict form).

Other Key Points and Reminders
• Always move slowly and smoothly (avoid speeding up as your muscles fatigue).

- Try to avoid dorsi-flexion (flexing your feet toward your knees and shins).
- Keep a loose grip on the handles (avoid any use of your hands and arms).
- Don't rest between repetitions or end a set until fully fatigued.

Seated or Supine Leg Press (Machine)

1. Select a weight that you're able to use for six to ten reps with strict form.
2. Adjust the seat back (forward or back) to allow for a full movement range.
3. Adjust the seat so there is minimal stress on your lower back (in general, the seat back angle should be about 45 degrees).
4. Lie back on the seat and place your hands very lightly on the grips.
5. Place your feet on the foot plate; they should be centered, with both feet flat.
6. Adjust your foot position; your feet should be roughly 12 inches apart. To direct more stress to your inner thighs, move your feet farther apart.
7. While keeping your buttocks and lower back in contact with the seat, extend your legs very slowly (don't hold your breath—exhale as you press).

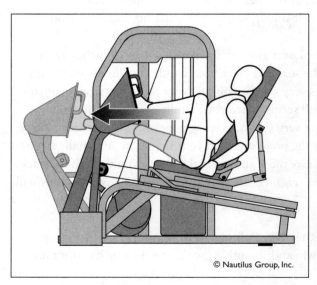

© Nautilus Group, Inc.

Figure 4.2
Seated Leg Press

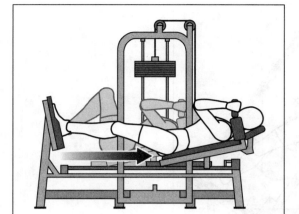

Figure 4.3
Supine Leg Press

8. Stop once your legs are extended to roughly three-fourths of a full movement range (past this point, there is minimal stress on your thighs and more on your knees).
9. Inhale and slowly lower the weight with your feet kept *flat* on the plate.
10. Lower the weight as much as you can without overstressing your knees. Also, stop if you find it hard to keep from arching your back.
11. Repeat until you reach failure (you can't perform any more reps with strict form).

Other Key Points and Reminders

- Don't bow or spread your knees—make sure you keep them aligned with your feet.
- To start the first rep without stressing your back, push down on your thighs with your hands.

45-Degree Hack Squat (Machine)

1. Select a weight that you're able to use for six to ten reps with strict form.
2. Assume the starting position, with your shoulders under the pads.
3. Center your feet on the foot plate, keeping them flat and pointed straight.
4. Adjust your foot position; your feet should be 1 to 2 feet apart.

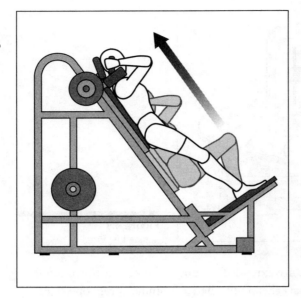

Figure 4.4
45-Degree Hack Squat

5. Reach up and grasp the handles, with your eyes focused straight ahead.
6. Release the weight by moving the handles out as far as you can.
7. While holding the handles lightly, very slowly lower the weight; your thighs should be roughly parallel to the platform when you stop. Never squat any lower than this or you'll risk injuring your knees.
8. While keeping your feet completely flat, slowly extend your legs.
9. Stop once your legs are extended to roughly three-fourths of a full movement range.
10. Lower the weight again promptly (you should not rest or pause at this point).
11. Repeat until you reach failure (you can't perform any more reps with strict form).

Other Key Points and Reminders

- At all times during this exercise keep your knees aligned with your feet. Don't ever bow or spread your knees, and make sure your feet stay flat.
- Keep your lower back flat against the back pad at all times.
- *Do not rest*—keep continuous tension on your thighs!

Seated Leg Curl (Machine)

1. Select a weight that you're able to use for six to ten reps with strict form.
2. Unlock and move the knee pad up to clear enough space for your legs.
3. Adjust the seat back and leg pad, using the guidelines on the machine. (With your legs in the starting position—straight, with your ankles on top of the pad—your knee joint should be strictly aligned with the centerpoint of the cam.)
4. Position your legs on the leg pad so that they're 1 to 6 inches apart.
5. Lower the knee pad and *lock* it once it touches the tops of your thighs.
6. Position your hands on the grips (above the knee pad or next to the seat).
7. Bend your legs very slowly, pointing your feet *away* from your shins.
8. Pause for one full second once your legs are maximally flexed.
9. Slowly extend your legs, without sliding forward or arching your back.
10. Repeat until you reach failure (do as many strict reps as you can).

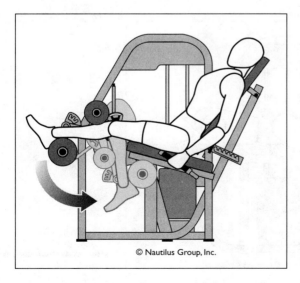

© Nautilus Group, Inc.

Figure 4.5
Seated Leg Curl

Other Key Points and Reminders

- Don't arch your back (this often occurs at the start and end of a rep).
- Don't hold your breath, lean forward, or pull on the handles (or seat) with your arms.
- Try not to use momentum—let your hamstrings move the weight!

Prone Leg Curl (Machine)

1. Select a weight that you're able to use for six to ten reps with strict form.
2. Adjust the leg pad (if possible) to accommodate your lower legs. Center the back of your ankle, above your heel, against the pad.
3. Assume a standing position between the leg pad and rear edge of the bench.
4. Assume a prone position (lie down on your stomach on top of the bench).
5. Slide forward or back until your knees are just off the edge of the bench.
6. Reach under the bench and place your hands very lightly on the grips.
7. Lift your legs until the backs of your ankles touch the pad.

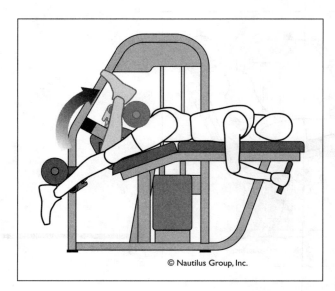

© Nautilus Group, Inc.

Figure 4.6
Prone Leg Curl

8. Tighten your buttocks, press your hips down, and slowly start lifting the weight. Don't lift your head or arch your back at any point during the lift.

9. Flex your legs as much as you can without lifting your hips from the bench. (If you can't avoid lifting your hips from the bench, you're using too much weight.)

10. Pause for one full second once your legs are maximally flexed.

11. Lower the weight very slowly, keeping your hips in contact with the bench.

12. Lower the weight as much as you can (without lifting your hips) and repeat.

Other Key Points and Reminders

- Use your hands only to keep yourself from moving forward or back.
- Resist the temptation to jerk the weight up—all lifts should be slow and controlled.
- Don't hold your breath, lift your hips from the bench, slide forward, or arch your back.
- Don't dorsi-flex (flex your feet toward your shins); instead, point them slightly *away*.

CALVES

Seated Calf Press (Machine)

1. Select a weight that you're able to use for eight to twelve reps with strict form.

2. Adjust the back of the seat to allow for a maximum movement range.

3. Assume a seated position with your feet centered on the plate.

4. With your feet flat on the foot plate, very slowly extend your legs. To take the stress off your lower back, push down on your thighs with your hands.

5. Move your feet down so that roughly two-thirds of each foot is below the plate.

6. Take your hands off your thighs and place them lightly on the grips.

7. Adjust your foot position; your feet should be 1 to 6 inches apart.

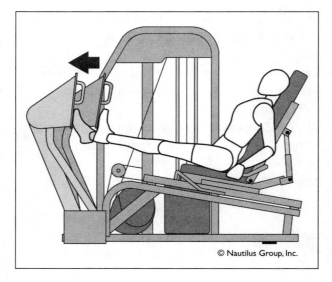

© Nautilus Group, Inc.

Figure 4.7
Seated Calf Press

8. With your legs completely extended, lower your heels beneath the plate. Move in a slow, controlled fashion, lowering your heels as much as you can.
9. Slowly press your feet forward, extending your feet as much as you can.
10. When your feet are pressed all the way forward, pause for one second and lower the weight.
11. Repeat until you reach failure (you can't perform any more reps with strict form).

Other Key Points and Reminders

- In general, keep your feet pointed straight (instead of in or out).
- Move through a *full* range of motion (if you can't, reduce the weight).
- Don't let your hips slide forward when performing this exercise.

Standing Calf Raise (Machine)

1. Pull the pin from the weight stack, so you are lifting just *one* plate.
2. Place your feet on the step and slide your shoulders under the pads.
3. Slowly lower your heels to the floor (with one-third of each foot on the step).

4. Lower your heels as much as you can (with your legs completely straight). If the moving part of the weight stack touches the part that stays in place, you need to move the shoulder pads down to allow for a full movement range.

5. Step off the machine and select a weight you can use for eight to twelve reps.

6. Slide your shoulders under the pads and place your feet on the step.

7. Stabilize your position by grasping the top or side of the machine.

8. Slide forward or back so that just the top third of your foot is on the step.

9. Adjust your foot position; your feet should be 1 to 6 inches apart.

10. Keep your feet pointed straight ahead (don't point your toes in or out).

11. Center your shoulders under the pads and slowly straighten your legs. Rise up on your toes as high as you can (without looking down at your feet).

12. Pause for one second when up on your toes, then slowly lower the weight.

13. Lower your heels as much as you can without sliding back on the step.

14. Repeat until you reach failure (you can't perform any more reps with strict form).

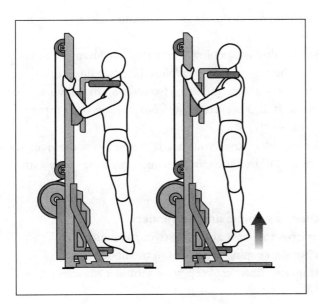

Figure 4.8
Standing Calf Raise

Other Key Points and Reminders

- Never bounce or jerk the weight up; make sure every rep is controlled.
- If you have (or have had) a knee problem, your knees should stay slightly bent.
- Always stay centered under the pads and try not to arch your back.
- Never wear old or worn footwear when you are using this type of machine. Your shoes should have a tread pattern that will give your feet some grip.

UPPER BACK

Wide-Grip Pulldown (Machine)

1. Select a weight that you're able to use for six to ten reps with strict form.
2. Sit down and adjust the leg pad (up or down) to make room for your legs. When locked in place, the leg pad should rest on the midpoint of your thighs.
3. Stand up and grasp the bar firmly with your palms turned away from your face. When gripping the bar, your hands should be about 3 to 4 feet apart.
4. Keep your arms straight as you slowly sit down and slide your thighs under the pads.
5. Pull the bar down very slowly, keeping your torso upright at all times.
6. Pull the bar down to the *top of your head*, and briefly pause at this point. This keeps your shoulders and arms from doing more work than your upper back. It also prevents you from moving your torso too far forward or back.
7. Extend your arms *completely* (over your head) as you lower the weight.
8. Repeat until you reach failure (you can't perform any more reps with strict form).

Other Key Points and Reminders

- If possible, face a mirror to assess and adjust your technique.
- Pull the bar down evenly, keeping it parallel to the floor.
- Don't tense your trapezius muscles; keep your shoulder muscles completely relaxed.

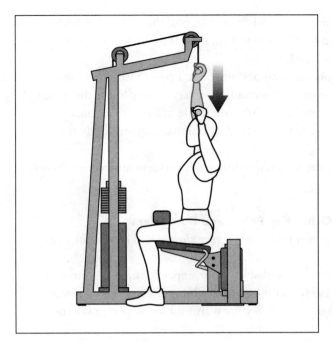

Figure 4.9
Wide-Grip Pulldown

- Pulling the bar to your *chin* requires greater use of your shoulders and arms. Pulling the bar to the *back of your neck* involves these groups even more.

Seated Cable Row (Machine)

1. Select a weight that you're able to use for six to ten reps with strict form.
2. Attach your choice of handle or bar to the cable clip on the machine. You will have many options to choose from, with varying lengths and grips. A wider grip will direct more stress to the outer part of your back, while a narrower grip will direct more stress to the area nearer your spine.
3. Face the weight stack, grasp the bar (or handle), and sit on the bench.
4. Place your feet on the foot plate, straighten your legs, and slide back on the bench. *Note:* Don't straighten your legs all the way—maintain a slight bend in your knees.
5. Ensure that your upper body stays perpendicular to the floor.

6. While maintaining an upright position, pull the handle (or bar) toward your waist. Move in a slow, fluid fashion, keeping your shoulders and neck relaxed.
7. Once the bar touches your abdomen (at a point just above your waist), pause for one full second, then very slowly lower the weight. *Note:* As you extend your arms, do not lean forward or back.
8. When your arms are *fully* extended, pull back again slowly (to raise the weight).
9. Repeat until you reach failure (you can't perform any more reps with strict form).

Other Key Points and Reminders

- Try not to use momentum—move very slowly and keep your back *straight!*
- In order to fully isolate and stress your upper back, keep your arms close to your torso (don't move your elbows away from your sides).
- Exhale as you pull the bar to your waist; inhale as you lower the weight.
- Move through a *full* range of motion (if you can't, reduce the weight).

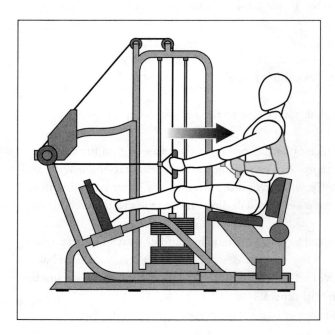

Figure 4.10
Seated Cable Row

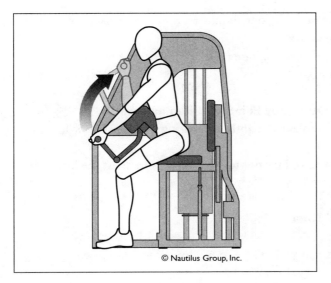

© Nautilus Group, Inc.

Figure 4.11
Seated Curl

BICEPS

Seated Curl (Machine)

1. Select a weight that you're able to use for six to ten reps with strict form.
2. Adjust the seat position based on the guidelines on the machine. In general, when seated upright (with your chest flush against the pad), your upper arms should be flush (and aligned) with the angled part of the pad.
3. Straddle the seat and grasp the handles, using a comfortable grip. If you grasp the angled part of the bar, there will be less stress on your wrists.
4. Align your elbow joints strictly with the centerpoint of the cam (on most machines, this point is marked with an arrow or red dot).
5. Pull the handles all the way back and sit upright on the seat (your elbows must stay strictly aligned with the centerpoint of the cam).
6. Keep your shoulders relaxed and straighten your arms as much as you can.
7. When your arms are fully extended, slowly begin to raise the weight.
8. Pause for one full second when your biceps are maximally flexed.
9. Lower the weight very slowly, keeping your wrists as straight as you

can. Also, don't hunch your shoulders, round your back, or slide back on the seat.

10. Repeat until you reach failure (you can't perform any more reps with strict form).

Other Key Points and Reminders

- Don't grip the handles too tightly (increasing the use of your forearms and wrists).
- Keep your feet flat and try not to use your legs to assist the lift.

Seated Dumbbell Curl

1. Select a weight that you're able to use for six to ten reps with strict form.
2. If possible, use an adjustable bench or seat with an upright back.
3. If possible, face a mirror to assess and adjust your technique.
4. Holding a dumbbell in each hand, position yourself on the seat.
5. Keeping your torso upright and your back flush against the seat, curl (lift) the dumbbells slowly, keeping your shoulders and neck relaxed.
6. Stop when your hands are level with the lowermost part of your chest. (If your upper arms start to move forward, you're lifting the weight too high.)
7. Lower the weight very slowly. Don't twist the dumbbells or bend your wrists.

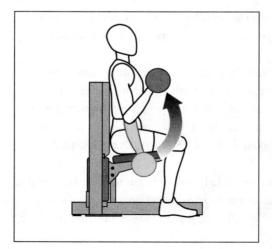

Figure 4.12
Seated Dumbbell Curl

8. Repeat until you reach failure (you can't perform any more reps with strict form).

Other Key Points and Reminders

- Make sure your movements are always controlled—do not jerk or swing the weight up.
- Your arms must be *fully* extended before you begin to raise the weight.

Seated Dumbbell Hammer Curl

1. Select a weight that you're able to use for six to ten reps with strict form.
2. If possible, use an adjustable bench or seat with an upright back.
3. If possible, face a mirror to assess and adjust your technique.
4. When seated, keep your arms straight and hold the weights parallel to your thighs.
5. Keeping your torso upright and your back flush against the seat, curl (lift) the dumbbells slowly, keeping your shoulders and neck relaxed.
6. Stop when your hands are level with the lowermost part of your chest. (If your upper arms start to move forward, you're lifting the weight too high.)
7. Lower the weight very slowly. Don't twist the dumbbells or bend your wrists.

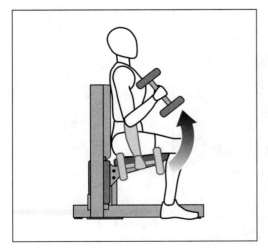

Figure 4.13
Seated Dumbbell Hammer Curl

8. Repeat until you reach failure (you can't perform any more reps with strict form).

Other Key Points and Reminders

- Maintain a "thumbs-up" position, both as you lift and lower the weight. Don't twist your wrists or change your grip at any point during the lift.
- Make certain your movements are always controlled—do not jerk or swing the weight up.
- Don't let your upper arms move forward or back while performing the lift.
- Your arms must be *fully* extended before you begin to lift the weight.

Standing Cable Curl (Machine)

1. Select a weight that you're able to use for six to ten reps with strict form.
2. To the cable, attach a bar that is either straight or slightly bent.
3. Squat with your back kept straight and grasp the bar with your palms facing up.

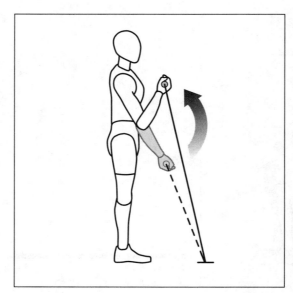

Figure 4.14
Standing Cable Curl

4. Stand up slowly, holding the bar with your arms completely straight.
5. Adjust the width of your grip so your hands are 8 to 12 inches apart.
6. Move forward or back until you are standing 2 to 3 feet from the stack. (You should be holding the bar about 6 to 12 inches away from your thighs.)
7. With your upper arms close to your torso, slowly begin to curl the weight.
8. Stop when your hands are strictly aligned with the lowermost part of your chest.
9. Extend your arms very slowly, keeping your arms against your sides.
10. Extend your arms completely before you begin another rep.
11. Repeat until you reach failure (you can't perform any more reps with strict form).

Other Key Points and Reminders

- Keep your neck and shoulders relaxed and your wrists as straight as you can.
- Don't arch your back or tuck your chin at any point during the lift.
- Steady your upper arms and hold them firmly against your sides.

CHEST

Vertical Chest Press (Machine)

1. Select a weight that you're able to use for six to ten reps with strict form.
2. Adjust your seat position based on the guidelines on the machine. Generally, when you are seated, the grips should align with your lower chest. On some machines, you may also adjust the height of the grips (or bar).
3. Press down on the foot bar with both feet and firmly grasp the grips.
4. Carefully take your feet off the bar and slowly extend your arms. Loosen your grip a little and keep your upper arms slightly raised.
5. Exhale as you straighten your arms, and try not to tense your face or neck.
6. When your arms are extended, *do not pause*; instead, promptly lower the weight.
7. Inhale, lower the weight as much as you can, and repeat the lift.

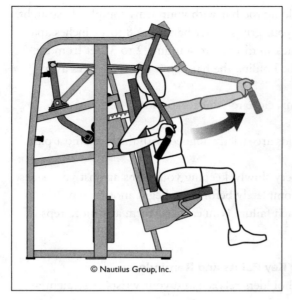

© Nautilus Group, Inc.

Figure 4.15
Vertical Chest Press

Don't raise your shoulders, arch your back, lean forward, or tense your neck.

8. Repeat until you reach failure (you can't perform any more reps with strict form).

Other Key Points and Reminders

- Try not to use momentum—don't perform rapid, explosive lifts.
- As you lower the weight, bring your hands back (past your chest) as much as you can.
- If you hear any rattling or clanging during a lift, you're moving too fast. (The machine may also need maintenance; ask the staff at your gym for help.)
- Press down on the foot bar immediately when you complete a set. Then let go of the grips and let your legs control the weight.

Pec Fly (Machine)

1. Select a weight that you're able to use for six to ten reps with strict form.

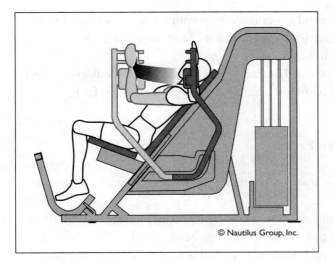

© Nautilus Group, Inc.

Figure 4.16
Pec Fly

2. Adjust the seat position based on the guidelines on the machine. (The seat adjustment will vary based on the type of machine you use.)
3. Sit and align your forearm with the center of one pad. Swing the pad forward until it's positioned in front of your shoulder or face. Then position your other arm behind the other pad.
4. Position your upper arms so they are parallel to the floor.
5. Assume a right-angle position with your upper and lower arms.
6. Start moving your arms together, pressing your forearms against the pads. (If there are handles on the machine, make sure you loosen your grip.) Try not to shrug your shoulders, tighten your neck, or arch your back.
7. When your arms are as close as possible, pause for one second, then lower the weight. Make sure you don't lean forward, raise your shoulders, or lift your hips.
8. Lower the weight as much as you can without arching your lower back.
9. Repeat until you reach failure (you can't perform any more reps with strict form).

Other Key Points and Reminders
• Keep your head aligned with your spine—don't bend or extend your neck.

- Keep your upper and lower back flush with the seat back at all times.
- Apply all the force with your forearms. Don't hold the grips tightly or push with your hands.
- If you have (or have had) an injury that involves your shoulders or chest, limit your range of motion, i.e., don't bring your arms too far back.

Free Weight Bench Press

1. Select a weight that you're able to use for six to ten reps with strict form.
2. Assume a supine position on the bench, with your feet on the floor.
3. Slide forward or back to center your head directly below the bar.
4. Grasp the bar and position your hands so they're about shoulder width apart.
5. Add about 3 to 6 inches to the width of your grip on each side.
6. Carefully lift the bar from the hooks or enlist a spotter for help.
7. Lower the weight very slowly, keeping your lower back *flat* on the bench.
8. Inhale as you lower the weight to the point where it gently touches your chest.
9. Exhale and slowly extend your arms, pressing up and back in a slight arc.
10. Keep your back and buttocks flat on the bench and feet flat on the floor.
11. When your arms are fully extended, slowly lower the weight and repeat.

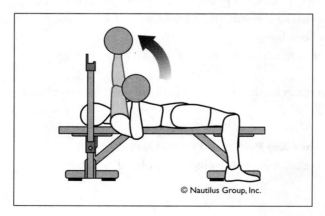

© Nautilus Group, Inc.

Figure 4.17
Free Weight Bench Press

12. Repeat until you reach failure (you can't perform any more reps with strict form).

Other Key Points and Reminders

- *Never* bounce the weight off your chest. Control the descent of the weight.
- Try not to raise your buttocks, arch your back, or hold your breath.
- Adjust your grip so your thumb is firmly secured around the bar. (Don't "cup" your thumb beneath the bar—this type of grip isn't safe.)
- Try not to use momentum—don't perform rapid, explosive lifts.
- Enlist the help of a spotter when you are using heavy weights.

TRICEPS

Cable Triceps Extension (Machine)

1. Select a weight that you're able to use for six to ten reps with strict form.

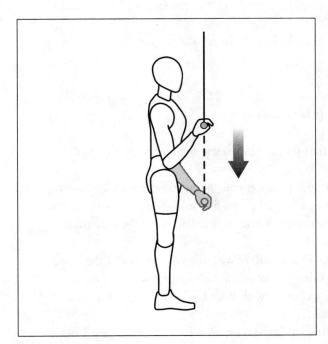

Figure 4.18
Cable Triceps Extension

2. Connect a straight or V-shaped bar (or a rope) to the top cable clip.
3. Face the machine and position yourself about 2 or 3 feet from the stack.
4. Grasp the bar or rope with your hands about 1 to 6 inches apart.
5. Pull down on the bar or rope and stop when your upper arms touch your ribs. Your arms should be flush with your torso, with your hands just below your chest.
6. With your neck and shoulders fully relaxed, slowly extend your arms. Your arms should be close to your body—try not to move them forward or back.
7. Pause for one full second once your arms are completely straight.
8. Lower the weight very slowly, without leaning forward or tensing your neck.
9. Stop once your hands are level with the lowermost part of your chest.
10. Perform as many strict reps as you can (don't force extra reps with poor form).

Other Key Points and Reminders
- Keep your wrists as straight as you can and try to relax your grip.
- Don't tuck your chin, turn your head to the side, or hyperextend your neck.
- Don't arch your back or lean forward. Keep your torso upright at all times.

Triceps Extension (Machine)

1. Select a weight that you're able to use for six to ten reps with strict form.
2. Straddle the seat and position your hands on the pads or hold the grips. If there are pads, make two fists and then turn your hands palms in. If there are grips, use the guidelines on the machine to position your hands.
3. Align your elbow joints strictly with the centerpoint of the cam. (*Note:* This point is often marked with an arrow or red dot.)
4. Assume a seated position, with your back straight and feet on the floor.
5. With your shoulders relaxed, very slowly straighten your arms as

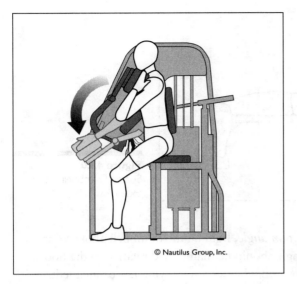

© Nautilus Group, Inc.

Figure 4.19
Triceps Extension (Machine)

much as you can. Make sure that the backs of your upper arms remain against the pad.

6. Pause for one full second once you've completely extended your arms.
7. Lower the weight very slowly, keeping your elbows firmly in place.
8. Repeat until you reach failure (you can't perform any more reps with strict form).

Other Key Points and Reminders

- Don't lift your buttocks off the seat at any time during the lift.
- Keep your shoulders completely relaxed. If you can't, reduce the weight.
- Always keep your upper arms in contact with the pad.

Supine (or Incline) Dumbbell Triceps Extension

1. Select a weight that you're able to use for six to ten reps with strict form.
2. Find a flat or adjustable bench and clear yourself plenty of space.
3. Grasp the dumbbell and lie (supine) on the flat or inclined bench.
4. Slide back until the top of your head is aligned with the edge of the bench.

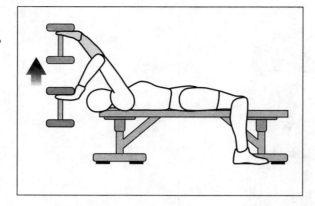

Figure 4.20
Supine Dumbbell Triceps
Extension

5. Position your arms *at an angle*, holding the dumbbell above your head (a 45-degree angle should be maintained relative to the floor). This is the proper position whether you're lying flat or inclined.

6. While holding your upper arms as close as you can to the sides of your head, lower the weight with your palms against the inside part of one end.

7. Extend your arms very slowly. Don't spread your elbows or move your hands.

8. Extend your arms as much as you can, then lower the weight and repeat.

9. Repeat until you reach failure (you can't perform any more reps with strict form).

Other Key Points and Reminders

- Keep your back flat against the bench at all times during the lift.
- Keep your upper arms stable—don't move them forward, back, or apart.
- Try not to raise your shoulders at any time when extending your arms.

Triceps Press (Machine)

1. Select a weight that you're able to use for six to ten reps with strict form.

2. Lower the seat just enough to allow for a maximum movement range.

3. Depending on what your goal is, move the handles forward or back. Your triceps will be stressed to a greater degree when the handles are back. When the handles are forward, there is more stress on your shoulders and lower chest.

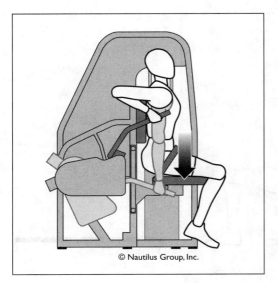

© Nautilus Group, Inc.

Figure 4.21
Triceps Press

4. Fasten the belt (to ensure that you stay in contact with the seat).
5. Reach back and grasp the handles (one at a time) with your palms facing in.
6. Straighten your arms as much as you can without tensing your shoulders or neck.
7. Pause for one full second, once you've fully extended your arms.
8. Lower the weight as much as you can without tensing your shoulders or neck.
9. Repeat until you reach failure (you can't perform any more reps with strict form).

Other Key Points and Reminders

- If you find yourself raising your shoulders, you are using too much weight.
- If you cannot extend your arms fully, you are using too much weight.

SHOULDERS

Seated Press (Machine)

1. Select a weight that you're able to use for six to ten reps with strict form.
2. Adjust the seat (up or down) to allow for a proper movement range.

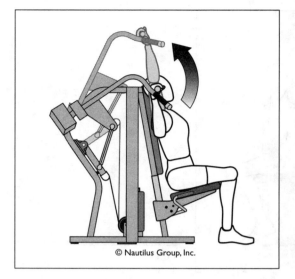

© Nautilus Group, Inc.

Figure 4.22
Seated Press

When you're seated, the grips should be level with, or just below, your ears.

3. Extend your arms very slowly, keeping your wrists as straight as you can.
4. When your arms are fully extended, lower the weight without a pause.
5. Lower the weight until your hands are slightly below your ears.
6. Repeat until you reach failure (you can't perform any more reps with strict form).

Other Key Points and Reminders

- To improve your grip, use training gloves designed for lifting weights.
- Exhale as you extend your arms, inhale as you lower the weight.
- Be careful not to arch your back—your spine should always be straight.

Seated Dumbbell Lateral Raise

1. Select a weight that you're able to use for six to ten reps with strict form.
2. If possible, face a mirror to assess and adjust your technique.
3. If possible, find a seat or bench that has an upright back.
4. Position yourself so your back is flush against the back of the seat.

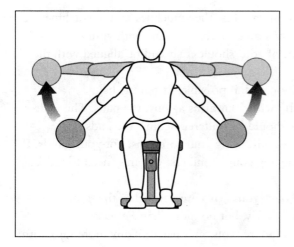

Figure 4.23
Seated Dumbbell Lateral Raise

5. With your arms slightly bent and your hands turned down, slowly raise the weights.
6. When the dumbbells reach shoulder level, your arms should be parallel to the floor. Pause at this point for one second, keeping your hands turned *slightly down.*
7. Lower the weights very slowly, with your arms very slightly bent.
8. Stop at the point where your shoulders begin to relax (about halfway down).
9. Repeat until you reach failure (you can't perform any more reps with strict form).

Other Key Points and Reminders

- Make sure that your arms are always raised perpendicular to your trunk. This will ensure that the medial part of your shoulder is maximally stressed.
- Never jerk or fling the weights up. All lifts should be slow and controlled.
- Be careful not to raise the weights too high when performing this lift. Stop when you reach shoulder level, pause, and slowly lower the weights.

Seated Lateral Raise (Machine)

1. Select a weight that you're able to use for six to ten reps with strict form.

2. Adjust your seat position based on the guidelines on the machine. Generally, when you are seated on the machine with your hands on the grips, the midpoint of your shoulder should be aligned with the dot on the cam.
3. Assume a seated position and, if possible, fasten the belt.
4. Grip the handles lightly with your arms against the pads. The widest part of your forearms should be centered against the pads.
5. Raise the weight very slowly, using your forearms, not your hands. If you find yourself shrugging your shoulders, you may need to reduce the weight.
6. Pause for one second once your arms are parallel to the floor.
7. Lower the weight very slowly, but no more than *halfway* down.
8. Repeat until you reach failure (you can't perform any more reps with strict form).

Other Key Points and Reminders

- Make sure all your movements are slow and controlled and your neck remains relaxed.
- Maintain a loose grip on the handles and keep your arms centered on the pads.

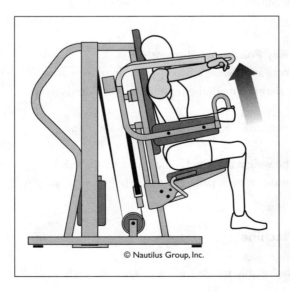

© Nautilus Group, Inc.

Figure 4.24
Seated Lateral Raise

Abdominal Crunch

1. Assume a supine position on an exercise mat or the floor.
2. Rest your feet on top of a chair, low bench, or exercise ball.
3. Ensure that your thighs are at 90 degrees (perpendicular) to the floor.
4. Cross your arms in front of your chest, or cradle your neck with your hands.
5. With your legs and feet close together, flatten your back and tighten your abs.
6. Begin to curl up very slowly, keeping your shoulders and neck relaxed. Keep your back flat, exhale, and tense your abs as hard as you can.
7. Pause for one full second when your abs are maximally tensed.
8. Inhale as you lower your shoulders. Stop when your shoulder blades touch the floor.
9. Repeat until you reach failure (you can't perform any more reps with strict form).

Other Key Points and Reminders

- Don't tuck your chin or extend your neck. Keep your neck fully relaxed.
- If you're able to do twelve reps (or more) maintaining perfect form, add some weight for resistance (hold it as high on your chest as you can).
- When you feel your shoulder blades touch the floor, don't let yourself relax—begin the next rep immediately. Pause when you're *up*, not down.
- Move in a slow, controlled fashion. Try not to rock or jerk yourself up.

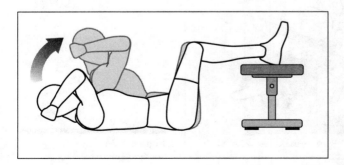

Figure 4.25
Abdominal Crunch

• Don't hold your breath or pull on the back of your neck as you curl yourself up.
• For a slightly different effect, try twisting your torso as you curl up. With your hands behind your head, rotate your right elbow toward your left knee. Pause in the up position, then repeat on the opposite side.

Abdominal Crunch (Machine—Seated or Supine)

1. Select a weight that you're able to use for eight to twelve reps with strict form.
2. Adjust your seat position based on the guidelines on the machine. In general, your navel should be aligned with the centerpoint of the cam.
3. Sit or lie down and place your feet behind or on top of the pads (the placement of your legs and feet will depend on the type of machine). If seated, place your feet behind the pads that are under the seat.
4. Place your hands lightly on the grips near your chest or beside your head, and position your chest, if appropriate, against the pad (or pads).
5. Position your feet, knees, and thighs so they are no more than 6 inches apart.

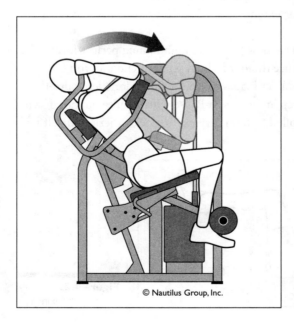

© Nautilus Group, Inc.

Figure 4.26
Seated Abdominal Crunch

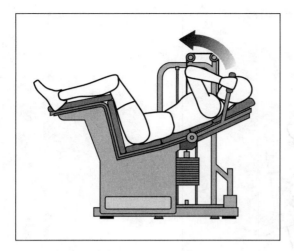

Figure 4.27
Supine Abdominal Crunch

6. Flatten your back, exhale, and flex your abdominals as you "crunch." Lift the weight with your abdominals instead of with your arms. Be sure to curl up very slowly, tensing your abs as hard as you can.
7. Pause for one full second when your abs are maximally flexed.
8. Inhale and lower the weight until the plates nearly touch the stack.
9. Repeat until you reach failure (you can't perform any more reps with strict form).

Other Key Points and Reminders
- If you're in the supine position, keep your head in contact with the pad.
- As you flex your abdominal muscles, flatten your back without lifting your hips.
- Only use weight that you're able to lift without having to use your arms.
- Try not to hold your breath at any time when performing this lift.

Knee Raise

1. Rest your forearms on the pads and position your hands on the grips.
2. With your knees and feet together and your back completely straight, lift your knees very slowly with your legs held slightly bent.
3. Tighten your abs and raise your knees as high as you can with strict form.
4. Pause for one full second before you begin to lower your legs.

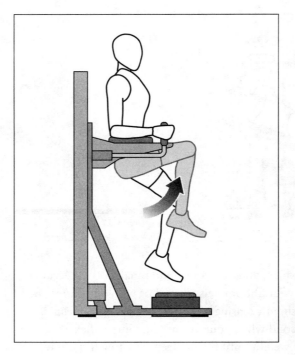

Figure 4.28
Knee Raise

5. Lower your legs with your knees kept bent, and stop about halfway down.
6. Repeat until you reach failure (you can't perform any more reps with strict form).

Other Key Points and Reminders
• Be careful not to arch your back or raise your legs too fast.

LOWER BACK

Lower Back Extension (Machine)

1. Pull the pin from the weight stack so you are lifting just *one* plate.
2. Adjust the foot plate up or down to allow your knees to stay bent.
3. Adjust the back pad, if possible, so it's aligned with your upper back.
4. Adjust the range mechanism to limit how far you extend your back.
5. Position yourself on the seat (adhere to the guidelines on the machine). Align your hip joint precisely with the centerpoint of the cam.

6. Press your back against the pad until you're upright on the seat.

7. Adjust and fasten the seat belt (or leg pads) to keep youself in place.

8. Slowly bend all the way forward until the plate rests against the stack.

9. Select a weight that you're able to use for six to ten reps with strict form.

10. Push down on your thighs with your hands and very slowly extend your back. Rest your hands on your abdomen once the weight begins to move.

11. Pause when you've *slightly* hyperextended your back, then lower the weight.

12. Repeat until you reach failure (you can't perform any more reps with strict form).

Other Key Points and Reminders

- Don't tuck your chin or extend your neck. Keep your head aligned with your spine.
- Try not to use your legs to assist—your back should do *all* the work.
- The weight should *gently* touch the stack—control the descent at all times.
- Be careful not to overextend your back if you're at risk. Ask your doctor or therapist to suggest an appropriate range.

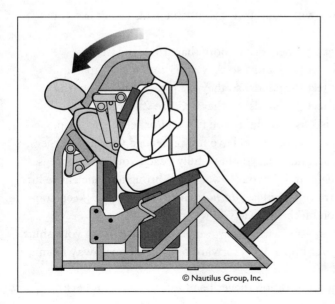

© Nautilus Group, Inc.

Figure 4.29
Lower Back Extension

- Don't hold your breath while performing this lift. Exhale as you lift the weight.
- Always perform this exercise at the end of your routine. Avoid fatiguing your lower back before doing other lifts.

ADDITIONAL EXERCISE OPTIONS

TECHNIQUE KEY

1. Never arch your lower back (make sure your spine is straight).
2. Try not to shrug your shoulders and/or tense your face and neck.
3. One-half range of motion.
4. Two-thirds range of motion.
5. Three-fourths range of motion.
6. Full range of motion.
7. Don't hold your breath (inhale as you lower, exhale as you lift).
8. Perform this movement *slowly* (don't use momentum—maintain control).
9. Keep your knees aligned with your feet (don't bow them in or out).
10. Keep your feet flat (don't raise your heels or push with the sides of your feet).
11. Apply the force with your arms against the pads (don't use your hands).
12. Keep your feet together (or no more than 1 inch apart).
13. Position your feet (or hands) so they are 3 to 6 inches apart.
14. Position your feet (or hands) so they are 6 to 12 inches apart.
15. Position your feet (or hands) so they are 1 to 2 feet apart.
16. Keep your wrists as straight as you can and/or relax your grip.
17. Hold for one second once you have fully extended your arms or legs.
18. Hold for one second once you have fully flexed your arms or legs.
19. Maintain a *slight* arch in your lower back throughout the entire lift.
20. As you perform this exercise, *do not* pause at any point (keep continuous tension on the muscle you want to stress).
21. Always position your feet so they are pointed away from your shins.
22. Don't move your upper arms forward or your elbows away from your sides.
23. Stay in an upright position (never bend forward or lean back).

24. Keep your legs straight (if possible) or maintain a *slight* bend in your knees.

For the following exercises, please refer to the technique key.

LOWER BODY

Quadriceps

- Free-Weight Squat: 5, 7, 8, 9, 10, 15, 19, 20
- Supine Squat (Machine): 1, 5, 7, 8, 9, 10, 14, 20
- Lunge (Dumbbell): 1, 5, 7, 8, 9, 10, 14, 20
- 45-Degree Leg Press (Machine): 1, 5, 7, 8, 9, 10, 14, 20

Hamstrings

- One-Legged Leg Curl (Machine): 6, 7, 8, 9, 14, 18, 19

Calves

- Seated Calf Raise: 1, 6, 7, 8, 9, 13, 17, 24

Inner Thigh

- Hip Adduction (Machine): 1, 2, 6, 7, 8, 18

Outer Thigh

- Hip Abduction (Machine): 1, 2, 6, 7, 8, 17

Buttocks

- Kneeling Hip Extension (Machine): 6, 7, 8, 9, 19

UPPER BODY

Upper Back

- Seated Row (Machine): 2, 6, 7, 8, 16, 18

Biceps

- Incline Dumbbell Curl: 2, 4, 7, 8, 16, 18, 22
- Incline/Prone Barbell Curl: 2, 5, 7, 8, 16, 18
- Standing Barbell Curl (Straight or EZ Curl Bar): 1, 2, 4, 7, 8, 15, 16, 18, 22, 23
- Preacher Curl (Barbell or Dumbbell): 1, 2, 4, 7, 8, 10, 14, 16, 18
- Cable Preacher Curl: 1, 2, 4, 7, 8, 10, 14, 16, 18

Lower Back

- Lower Back Hyperextension (Roman Chair): 4, 7, 8, 14, 18

Chest

- Incline Bench Press (Barbell): 1, 6, 7, 8, 16, 20
- Incline Chest Press (Machine): 1, 6, 7, 8, 16, 20
- Decline Bench Press (Barbell): 1, 6, 7, 8, 16, 20
- Parallel Dips: 6, 7, 8, 16, 17, 19
- Parallel Dips (Assisted/Machine): 6, 7, 8, 16, 17, 19
- Supine Dumbbell Fly: 1, 2, 5, 7, 8, 16, 20
- Supine Cable Fly: 1, 2, 5, 7, 8, 16, 20
- Incline Cable Fly: 1, 2, 5, 7, 8, 16, 20
- Standing Cable Crossover: 1, 2, 5, 7, 8, 15, 16, 18

Triceps

- Triceps Push-Up (Torso Elevated, Feet on Floor): 1, 2, 6, 7, 8, 13, 20
- Seated Triceps Extension (Dumbbell): 1, 2, 6, 7, 8, 17

- Seated Triceps Extension (Barbell): 1, 2, 6, 7, 8, 14, 17
- Reverse Triceps Push-Up (Feet on Floor or Elevated, Hands on Bench): 6, 7, 8, 17

Forearms

- Seated Wrist Curl (Barbell): 2, 6, 7, 8, 13, 18, 22
- Seated Wrist Curl (Machine): 2, 6, 7, 8, 13, 18, 22

Abdominals

- Sit-ups: 1, 5, 7, 8, 9, 14, 20

Trapezius

- Shoulder Shrug (Machine): 1, 6, 7, 8, 18, 23
- Shoulder Shrug (Barbell): 1, 6, 7, 8, 14, 18, 23

CHAPTER FIVE

THE STRETCHES

I'm not into working out. My philosophy: No pain, no pain.
CAROL LEIFER

Some people think if they exercise right or stretch in a certain way they will shrink or elongate their muscles, giving them longer and thinner limbs. If you think this, too, it's important for you to know that this isn't true. Pilates can't do it, yoga can't do it, neither can using a rack—the truth is that no special movements can lengthen or shrink your muscles and bones. All right, I'll admit that technically, yes, you can lengthen your *muscles* a bit, but in this case "a bit" means a miniscule change—a change that's too tiny to see. So if you're convinced that your muscles look longer or thinner because of some stretch, you're probably either imagining things or have recently lost some weight. I don't say this to discourage you from taking the time to stretch, but rather so that you will understand what stretching can truly do.

WHAT STRETCHING DOES

- Stretching helps make your muscles much less likely to cramp or tear.
- Stretching can help increase your range of motion when lifting a weight.
- Stretching makes you more flexible (which can improve your performance in sports).
- Stretching can help you perform your everyday tasks with greater ease.

THE WRONG WAY TO STRETCH

- Bouncing, jerking, or pulsing can tear muscle fibers and injure joints. This often creates scar tissue, both in your muscles *and* your joints.

THE RIGHT WAY TO STRETCH

- Always ensure that your muscles are warm before you attempt to stretch. (Generally, walking or riding a bike for five to ten minutes will do.)
- For best results—and to lessen the risk to your muscles, spine, and joints —only perform *static* stretches, *held* at the point of maximum stretch.
- According to studies, a stretch works best with a *thirty*-second hold. Holding a stretch any longer than this isn't apt to improve your result.
- Rather than do a sequence of stretches before you begin your routine, do *one* stretch before you train individual muscle groups. For example, stretch your shoulders prior to doing a seated press. Or just before doing calf raises, take some time to stretch your calves. If ten or more minutes pass before you work a particular group, the muscles you stretched before your routine may no longer be relaxed.
- *Flex* the muscle you're targeting right before you begin each stretch. Hold for at least ten seconds and then promptly begin your stretch.
- Exhale as you move into a stretch and remember to take it *slow*!

QUADRICEPS

Standing Quad Stretch

1. Stand and place your right hand on a wall (or an object that won't move).
2. Lift your right foot toward the back of your thigh and grasp it with your left hand.
3. Slowly pull your foot as close as you can to the back of your thigh.
4. Maintain a *thirty*-second hold at the point of maximum stretch. (*Note:* This stretch should be *static*, which means you should never pulse or bounce).
5. Wait for ten seconds, then repeat the stretch with the opposite leg.

Other Key Points and Reminders

- Without leaning forward, lift your knee farther back to increase your stretch. Be careful not to arch your back or lean to the opposite side.
- Don't overstress your knee joint—stop if you feel discomfort or strain.
- You'll be less apt to lose your balance if you grasp a post or bar.

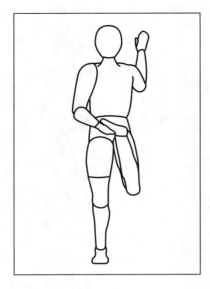

Figure 5.1
Standing Quad Stretch

HAMSTRINGS

Hamstring Stretch

1. Assume a seated position, keeping one leg completely straight.
2. Place the sole of your opposite foot against your inner thigh.
3. Keep your back straight, exhale, and move your chest *slowly* toward your straight leg. Keep your torso centered over your thigh throughout the stretch.
4. Hold for *thirty* seconds at the point of maximum stretch.
5. Raise your torso slowly and repeat with the opposite leg.

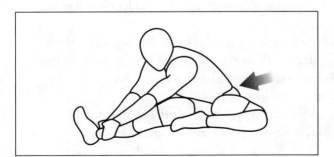

Figure 5.2
Hamstring Stretch

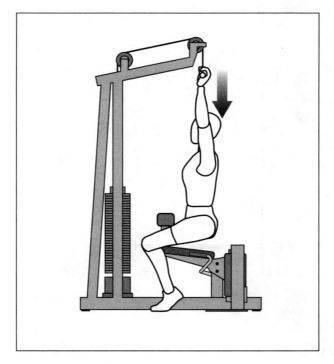

Figure 5.3
Lat Stretch

UPPER BACK

Lat (Upper Back) Stretch

1. Face a chin-up bar or a bar attached to a pulldown machine. If performing this stretch on a pulldown machine, put the pin at the bottom of the stack.
2. Grasp the bar with your hands spaced slightly wider than shoulder width.
3. Allow your body to hang from the bar (your feet can be on the floor). For a maximum stretch, allow the *full* weight of your body to hang from the bar. For a more relaxed stretch, support your weight by keeping your feet on the floor.
4. Hold for *thirty* seconds at the point of maximum stretch.
5. Repeat, if you like, with your hands either closer together or farther apart.

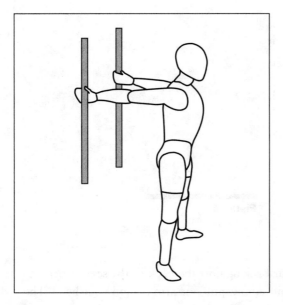

Figure 5.4
Chest Stretch

CHEST

Chest Stretch

1. With both arms straight, held out to your sides, and parallel to the floor, place your forearms or hands against a door frame or two posts. (If you're working out in a gym, you can do this stretch between machines.)
2. Slowly walk or lean forward, keeping your arms completely straight.
3. Hold for *thirty* seconds at the point of maximum stretch.

Other Key Points and Reminders

- To feel this stretch in different ways, move your arms up or down.

TRICEPS

Triceps Stretch

1. Assume a seated position on a seat or bench with a back.

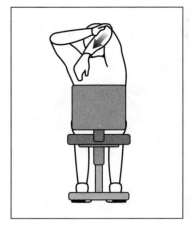

Figure 5.5
Triceps Stretch

2. Sit up straight with your back against the back of the seat or bench.
3. With a firm grasp of your elbow, pull one arm behind your head. The arm you're pulling behind your head is the one you're trying to stretch.
4. Pull the arm that you're stretching behind your head as much as you can. Hold it for thirty seconds at the point of maximum stretch.
5. Repeat with the opposite arm while keeping your lower back flush with the seat.

SHOULDERS

Shoulder Stretch

1. Kneel on the floor and place your hands on top of a bench or chair.
2. Move away from the bench or chair until your arms are straight.

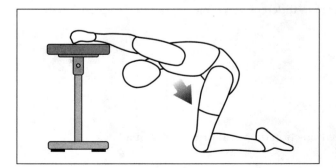

Figure 5.6
Shoulder Stretch

3. With both arms straight, slowly lower your torso toward the floor.
4. Hold for *thirty* seconds at the point of maximum stretch.

Other Key Points and Reminders

- Vary the distance between your hands to change the effect of this stretch.

CALVES

Standing Calf Stretch

1. Face a wall or anything you can lean against or grasp. Place your hands against the wall or grasp a bar or post.
2. Move the leg you're stretching *back* about 3 to 4 feet from your hands.
3. While keeping your forward leg bent at the knee and your back leg perfectly straight, press the heel of your back foot down so it's *flat* on the ground or floor. Make sure that during this stretch this foot remains pointed straight ahead.
4. Press your hips toward the wall (or whatever you've grasped) without lifting your heel. You can raise the heel of your forward foot (it does not have to be kept flat).

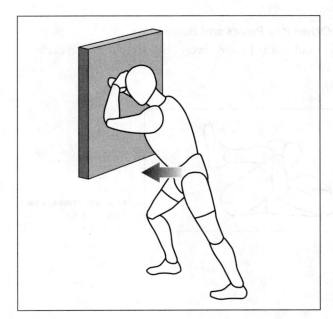

Figure 5.7
Standing Calf Stretch

5. Move your hips as close to the wall as you can without lifting your heel.
6. Maintain a *thirty*-second hold at the point of maximum stretch.
7. Wait for at least ten seconds, then repeat with the opposite leg.

Other Key Points and Reminders

- Experiment with the placement of your feet to increase your stretch (for example, try moving your feet a little farther away from the wall).
- For a good variation (to shift the stress to the lower part of your calves), bend the back leg at the knee, while keeping your heel completely flat (you will feel the stretch in the Achilles tendon area of your calf). Make sure your foot is pointed straight, and don't bow or spread your knees.

LOWER BACK

Lower Back Stretch

1. Assume a supine position and slowly raise one knee to your chest.
2. Slowly raise the opposite knee and hold both knees with your hands.
3. Slowly pull both knees as close as possible to your chest.
4. Hold for *thirty* seconds at the point of maximum stretch.

Other Key Points and Reminders

- Don't raise your head toward your knees. Your shoulders and neck should be fully relaxed.

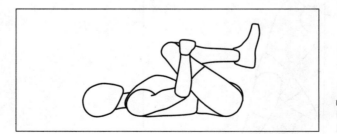

Figure 5.8
Lower Back Stretch

CHAPTER SIX

NUTRITIONAL GUIDELINES

You better cut that pizza into four slices
because I don't think I'm hungry enough to eat eight!
                                        YOGI BERRA

Now I am going to reveal to you the secret to losing weight. Are you ready? *The key to losing weight is finding out why you can't.* This probably sounds like something Yogi would say, but let me explain.

Before any diet, no matter how perfect it is, can help you lose weight, you must overcome the hidden blocks that will keep you from staying on course (or from achieving your goals, should you actually manage to stay with the plan). Whether it's a food allergy, yeast overgrowth, or PMS, unless stumbling blocks are unearthed and pulled up at their roots, your diet will fail. Here are some of the UFOs that can keep you from losing weight:

- Food allergies or intolerances, such as lactose, yeast, or wheat
- Snack amnesia (forgetting how much, and how often, you eat during the day)
- Hypothyroidism (underactive thyroid gland)
- Premenstrual syndrome (mood swings often cause women to overeat)
- Depression (you eat out of boredom or to get an emotional boost)
- Being on the wrong birth control pill or wrong combination of drugs
- Low levels of testosterone and/or DHEA
- Excessive consumption of alcohol (more than four or five drinks a week)
- Poor body image (may cause you to binge or overeat unhealthy foods)
- Improper food combining (fruits and vegetables are a bad mix)
- Diet misconceptions ("If I eat rice cakes, I'll lose weight.")

- Social and/or work-related gatherings and events
- Candidiasis (yeast overgrowth) (see page 45)
- Energy blocks/reversals (see Chapter Seven, page 209)
- Insulin instability (see page 71)

Okay, so what if you do address your weight-loss UFOs, and the diet you're on still doesn't work and you fail to lose much weight? *Now* is the time to ask yourself, "Am I on the right diet or not?" But how can you know, with so much conflicting advice being bandied about? Indeed, this can be a problem, but I'll explain how it can be solved: Quite simply, you must choose your diet based on your weight-loss UFOs! If the plan you're on, for example, accounts for your state of digestive health, it's bound to work considerably better for you than plans that don't. Or, if you have food allergies (or can't tolerate certain foods), obviously your diet shouldn't include the offending foods.

In general, I've found that people do best with one of three different plans. Consider the following guidelines for choosing the one that will serve you best:

- If insulin instability is on your top ten UFO list, observe the nutritional guidelines that are outlined in Plan B. (If candidiasis is also on your list, then use Plan C.)
- If your top ten UFO list includes candidiasis (yeast overgrowth), observe the nutritional guidelines that are outlined in Plan C.
- If neither of the above is on your top ten UFO list, observe the nutritional guidelines that are outlined in Plan A.

Plan A starts on page 186, Plan B on page 193, and Plan C on page 199.

BASIC NUTRITIONAL GUIDELINES

1. The optimum rate of weight loss is 1 to 2 pounds a week. If you lose any more than this, you're apt to lose muscle as well as fat.
2. Shoot for eight, or at least six, glasses of water every day.
3. If possible, eat smaller meals at regular intervals during the day. For example, instead of three large meals, have three smaller meals with three snacks.
   Example: Breakfast, 7 A.M.; midmorning snack, 9:30 A.M.; lunch, 12 P.M.; midafternoon snack, 3 P.M.; dinner, 6:30 P.M.; evening snack, 9:30 P.M.

4. To eliminate energy swings that cause fatigue throughout the day, be sure to include some type of protein source with your largest meals.

5. To prevent snack amnesia, "portion distortion," and going too long between meals, keep a food log to record your eating pattern throughout the day. (Refer to the sample food log on page 207.)

SUPPLEMENTS

Here are some things to bear in mind when considering supplement use:

1. *Most people who use supplements shoot in the dark and usually miss.* At the very least, supplement use should be based on a well-informed guess, i.e., it should target deficiencies, confirmed with reliable tests. Blood tests often can help to determine where your deficiencies lie.

2. *Some supplements, taken together, have an adverse or negating effect.* For example, it may be best to avoid unbuffered vitamin C, as it actually blocks the absorption of certain supplements and/or drugs.*

3. *People vary considerably when it comes to supplement needs.* Allow for some trial and error to assess your specific needs. (Monitor overdose symptoms and interactions by keeping a log.)

4. *If you notice unusual side effects, such as flushing, headaches, and fatigue, be sure to call your physician and put a hold on your supplement use.* A niacin flush, for example, can often result from an overdose, and excessive doses of vitamins A, D, and E can cause problems as well (these are fat-soluble vitamins, which at high doses can cause you harm).

5. *People are much too trusting when it comes to supplement claims.* For example, to find alternative ways to help cancer patients heal, the National Cancer Institute did research on supplement use. The results of the study suggested that supplement use does not always help, and even has the potential to cause a lot more harm than good. In another study, the Institute found that when vitamins fail to work it may be because they only help if ingested directly through food. Get a thumbs-up from your doctor before you start taking anything new, and bear in mind that at first it is best to take less than the label suggests.

---

* For more information on adverse interactions, check out *Nutrition Almanac* (5th Ed.), by Lavon J. Dunne, McGraw-Hill, 2001.

6. *Supplements should be allergen-free and without additives or dyes.* Allergic responses include hot flashes, rashes, gas, and fatigue. Be sure to check labels carefully and don't get attached to brand names. Sometimes, lesser-known companies offer quality products, too!

7. *A multivitamin may provide some nutrients that you lack, such as magnesium, folic acid, zinc, and omega-3.*

8. *A supplement is more likely to benefit you if it's time-released.* Otherwise, only a very small part of what you consume may be used.

9. *Don't trust studies that haven't been reproduced by an unbiased source.* Translation: You should take whatever you hear with a grain of salt. Studies are often fudged or skewed to support a company's claims, so when something sounds too good to be true, don't be surprised if it is.

A FORMULA FOR DETERMINING DAILY CALORIC INTAKE FOR WEIGHT LOSS— THE HARRIS-BENEDICT EQUATION

1. Multiply your weight (in pounds) by 0.453593.
   The result will be your body weight in kilograms (kg).
   Example: 195 lbs. × 0.453593 = 88.45 kg

2. Multiply your height (in inches) by 2.54.
   The result will be your height in centimeters (cm).
   Example: 70 inches × 2.54 = 177.8 cm

3. Use the following formula to determine your basal energy expenditure (BEE):

   MALE
   66 + (13.7 × weight in kg) + (5 × height in cm) − (6.8 × your age in years) = your BEE

   Example: A 195-pound man would weigh 88.45 kilograms. If he was 5'10" tall, he would have a height of 177.8 centimeters. If he was 37 years old, his equation would look like this:

   66 + (13.7 × 88.45) + (5 × 177.8) − (6.8 × 37) =
   66 + 1,211.77 + 889 − 251.6 = 1,915.17
   BEE = 1,915 calories per day

FEMALE
655 + (9.6 × weight in kg) + (1.7 × height in cm) − (4.7 × your age in years) = your BEE

Example: A 150-pound woman would weigh 68 kilograms. If she was 5'5" tall, she would have a height of 165 centimeters. If she was 40 years old, her equation would look like this:

655 + (9.6 × 68) + (1.7 × 165) − (4.7 × 40) =
655 + 652.8 + 280.5 − 188 = 1,400
BEE = 1,400 calories per day

4. Multiply your BEE by your activity rating:

- 1.25 if you're sedentary (little or no exercise)
- 1.5 if you're moderately active (you train two to three times a week)
- 1.75 if you're active (you train three or more times a week)

The result is the number of calories needed each day to maintain your weight.

Example: Using the first example, if you were a very active 37-year-old male, you would multiply your BEE (1,915 calories) × 1.75. The result would be 3,351 calories per day.

5. To determine your daily caloric intake for weight loss, subtract (from your daily caloric intake for weight maintenance):

- 500 (if you weigh less than 130 pounds)
- 1,000 (if you weigh between 130 and 230 pounds)
- 1,500 (if you weigh more than 230 pounds)

In general, this will allow for a loss of 1 to 2 pounds a week. Please note that 1,200 calories should be the least you consume per day (regardless of what the equation suggests your daily intake should be).

Example: Using the above example, you would subtract 1,000 from 3,351. The result would be 2,351 calories per day.

6. If you lose more than 2 pounds a week, *add* four servings to your plan. If you lose *less* than a pound, *subtract* four servings from your plan or increase your activity level (based on the guidelines in this book).

PLAN A—GENERAL

25 to 30 percent protein
50 percent complex carbohydrates
20 to 25 percent poly or monounsaturated (omega-3 rich) fat

For serving sizes, see page 189.

1,200 CALORIES PER DAY

Breakfast
1 serving grains and starches
1 serving protein
1 serving milk and dairy
1 serving fat

Snack
1 serving fruit

Lunch
1 serving vegetables
2 servings grains and starches
1 serving protein
1 serving fat

Snack
1 serving protein or fruit

Dinner
1 serving vegetables
2 servings protein
1 serving fat

Snack
>   1 serving protein or fruit

Total: 16 servings

1,500 CALORIES PER DAY

Breakfast
>   2 servings grains and starches
>   1 serving protein
>   1 serving milk and dairy
>   1 serving fat

Snack
>   1 serving fruit

Lunch
>   1 serving vegetables
>   2 servings grains and starches
>   2 servings protein
>   1 serving fat

Snack
>   1 serving protein or fruit

Dinner
>   2 servings vegetables
>   2 servings protein
>   1 serving grains and starches
>   1 serving fat

Snack
>   1 serving protein or fruit

Total: 20 servings

1,800 CALORIES PER DAY

Breakfast
1 serving fruit
2 servings grains and starches
2 servings protein
1 serving milk and dairy
1 serving fat

Snack
1 serving fruit

Lunch
2 servings vegetables
2 servings grains and starches
2 servings protein
1 serving fat

Snack
1 serving protein or fruit

Dinner
2 servings vegetables
2 servings protein
2 servings grains and starches
1 serving fat

Snack
1 serving protein or fruit

Total: 24 servings

2,100 CALORIES PER DAY

Breakfast
1 serving fruit
2 servings grains and starches

2 servings protein
2 servings milk and dairy
1 serving fat

Snack
1 serving fruit

Lunch
2 servings vegetables
2 servings grains and starches
3 servings protein
1 serving fat

Snack
1 serving protein or fruit

Dinner
3 servings vegetables
3 servings protein
2 servings grains and starches
1 serving fat

Snack
1 serving protein or fruit

Total: 28 servings

SERVING SIZES

Fruit
Apple–1 small
Apricots–2 medium
Banana–½ small
Berries–1 cup
Cantaloupe–¼ medium
Cherries–10 large
Grapefruit–½ small

Grapes–½ cup
Honeydew melon–⅛ medium
Orange–1 small
Orange juice–½ cup
Peach–1 medium
Pineapple–½ cup
Plums and prunes–2 medium
Tangerine–1 large
Tomato juice–1 cup
Unsweetened cranberries–as desired
Watermelon–1 cup

Vegetables

Starred vegetables (*): One serving equals ½ cup.
Unstarred vegetables: Use as desired.

Alfalfa sprouts
Artichokes
Asparagus
Broccoli
Brussels sprouts
Cabbage
Carrots*
Cauliflower
Celery
Chickpeas*
Corn*
Cucumbers
Dark green leafy vegetables (chard, spinach)
Eggplant
Green beans
Green peas*
Green peppers
Mushrooms
Okra
Onions*
Parsnips*
Pumpkin*

Radishes
Red peppers
Rutabagas*
Salad vegetables (chicory, endive, lettuce, parsley, watercress)
Spinach
String beans
Summer squash
Tomatoes
Turnips*
Wax beans
Winter squash*
Zucchini*

Grains and Starches

Whole grain bread–1 slice
Cereal, cooked–½ cup
Cereal, dry flake–¾ cup
Popcorn, popped–1 cup
Potatoes, baked or broiled–1 small
Potatoes, mashed–½ cup
Potatoes, sweet–½ cup or ½ small
Brown rice, cooked–½ cup
Pasta, cooked–½ cup
Wheat germ–2 rounded tablespoons

Protein

Egg–1 medium
Egg beaters or egg whites–¼ cup
Beans (soybeans, lentils)–1 cup
Soy meat/burger–2-ounce patty
Red meat (beef)[†]–2 ounces
Sesame seeds–1½ tablespoons
Sunflower seeds–1½ tablespoons
Sea bass–2 ounces
Cod–3 ounces
Haddock–3 ounces

[†] Limit to once a week (leanest cut).

Halibut–3 ounces
Lobster–1 ounce
Mackerel–3 ounces
Salmon–3 ounces
Scallops–2 ounces
Shrimp–2 ounces
Red snapper–3 ounces
Swordfish–2 ounces
Trout–2 ounces
Tuna (steak)–1 ounce
Tuna, canned (water packed)–1 ounce
Chicken (white meat, skinless, free-range)–2 ounces
Turkey (white meat, skinless, free-range)–2 ounces
Soymilk–¾ cup
Protein powder–⅓ ounce
Tofu (firm)–3 ounces

Milk and Dairy

Nonfat or skim milk–1 cup
Milk (1% fat)–¾ cup
Nonfat yogurt (unsweetened)–1 cup
Low-fat yogurt (unsweetened)–¾ cup
Evaporated skim milk–½ cup
Skim milk (dry powder)–¼ cup
Cottage cheese (low-fat)–¼ cup
Cheese (American or Swiss)–2-ounce slice

Fat

Margarine (polyunsaturated)–1 teaspoon
Diet margarine–2 teaspoons
Oil-type salad dressing–1 tablespoon
Mayonnaise–1 teaspoon
Soy mayonnaise–1½ teaspoons
Diet mayonnaise–1½ teaspoons
Vegetable oil–1 teaspoon
Olives–5 small
Olive oil–¾ teaspoon
Avocado–⅛ medium

PLAN B—INSULIN INSTABILITY

30 percent protein

45 to 50 percent low-glycemic carbohydrates

20 to 25 percent poly or monounsaturated (omega-3 rich) fat

For serving sizes, see page 196.

1,200 CALORIES PER DAY

Breakfast

1 serving grains and starches

1 serving protein

1 serving milk and dairy

1 serving fat

Snack

1 serving fruit

Lunch

1 serving vegetables

2 servings grains and starches

2 servings protein

Snack

1 serving protein or fruit

Dinner

1 serving vegetables

2 servings protein

1 serving fat

Snack

1 serving protein or fruit

Total: 16 servings

1,500 CALORIES PER DAY

Breakfast
1 serving grains and starches
2 servings protein
1 serving milk and dairy
1 serving fat

Snack
1 serving fruit

Lunch
1 serving vegetables
2 servings grains and starches
2 servings protein
1 serving fat

Snack
1 serving protein or fruit

Dinner
2 servings vegetables
2 servings protein
1 serving grains and starches
1 serving fat

Snack
1 serving protein or fruit

Total: 20 servings

1,800 CALORIES PER DAY

Breakfast
3 servings grains and starches
2 servings protein
1 serving milk and dairy
1 serving fat

Snack

1 serving fruit

Lunch

2 servings vegetables
2 servings grains and starches
2 servings protein
1 serving fat

Snack

1 serving protein or fruit

Dinner

2 servings vegetables
2 servings protein
2 servings grains and starches
1 serving fat

Snack

1 serving protein or fruit

Total: 24 servings

2,100 CALORIES PER DAY

Breakfast

3 servings grains and starches
2 servings protein
2 servings milk and dairy
1 serving fat

Snack

1 serving fruit

Lunch

3 servings vegetables
2 servings grains and starches

3 servings protein
1 serving fat

Snack
1 serving protein or fruit

Dinner
2 servings vegetables
3 servings protein
2 servings grains and starches
1 serving fat

Snack
1 serving protein or fruit

Total: 28 servings

FOODS TO AVOID OR EAT SPARINGLY (HIGH-GLYCEMIC)

Extremely high: puffed rice, cornflakes, millet, instant rice, instant potato, French bread, cooked parsnips, baked potato, cooked carrots, fava beans, white bread, foods containing simple sugars (maltose, glucose, and honey)

High: wheat bread, grape nuts, tortilla chips, shredded wheat, muesli, rye bread, brown rice, oats, sweet corn, white rice, mashed potatoes, boiled potato, apricots, raisins, bananas, papaya, mango, corn chips, candy, crackers, cookies, pastry, low-fat ice cream

Moderately high: buckwheat, All-Bran, spaghetti, yams, sweet potato, green peas, baked beans, kidney beans, fruit cocktail, grapefruit juice, orange juice, pineapple juice, canned pears, grapes, potato chips, sponge cake

SERVING SIZES

Fruit
Apple–1 small
Berries–1 cup
Cantaloupe–¼ medium
Cherries–10 large

Grapefruit–½ small
Honeydew melon–⅛ medium
Orange–1 small
Peach–1 medium
Pineapple–½ cup
Plums–2 medium
Watermelon–1 cup

Vegetables

Starred vegetables (*): One serving equals ½ cup.
Unstarred vegetables: Use as desired.

Alfalfa sprouts
Artichokes
Asparagus
Broccoli
Brussels sprouts
Cabbage
Cauliflower
Celery
Chickpeas*
Cucumbers
Dark green leafy vegetables (chard, spinach)
Eggplant
Green beans
Green peppers
Mushrooms
Okra
Onions*
Parsnips*
Pumpkin*
Radishes
Red peppers
Rutabagas*
Salad vegetables (chicory, endive, lettuce, parsley, watercress)
Spinach
String beans
Summer squash
Tomatoes
Turnips*

Wax beans
Winter squash*
Zucchini*

Grains and Starches

Oatmeal (slow-cooking)–⅓ cup cooked (½ ounce dry)
Barley (dry)–½ tablespoon
Rye bread–1 slice
Wheat germ–2 rounded tablespoons

Protein

Egg–1 medium
Egg beaters or egg whites–¼ cup
Beans (soybeans, lentils)–1 cup
Soy meat/burger–2-ounce patty
Red meat (beef)*–2 ounces
Sesame seeds–1½ tablespoons
Sunflower seeds–1½ tablespoons
Sea bass–2 ounces
Cod–3 ounces
Haddock–3 ounces
Halibut–3 ounces
Lobster–1 ounce
Mackerel–3 ounces
Salmon–3 ounces
Scallops–2 ounces
Shrimp–2 ounces
Red snapper–3 ounces
Swordfish–2 ounces
Trout–2 ounces
Tuna (steak)–1 ounce
Tuna, canned (water packed)–1 ounce
Chicken (white meat, skinless, free-range)–2 ounces
Turkey (white meat, skinless, free-range)–2 ounces
Soymilk–¾ cup
Protein powder–⅓ ounce
Tofu (firm)–3 ounces

*Limit to once a week (leanest cut).

Milk and Dairy

Nonfat or skim milk–1 cup
Milk (1% fat)–¾ cup
Skim milk (dry powder)–¼ cup
Cottage cheese (low-fat)–¼ cup
Cheese (American or Swiss)–2-ounce slice

Fat

Almond butter–⅓ teaspoon
Almonds–4 medium
Avocado–⅛ medium
Canola oil–½ teaspoon
Guacamole–1 tablespoon
Olive oil–¾ teaspoon
Olive oil and vinegar dressing–⅓ teaspoon olive oil and
    ⅔ teaspoon vinegar
Olives–5 small
Peanut butter (natural)–½ teaspoon
Peanut oil–⅓ teaspoon
Peanuts–6 medium
Margarine (polyunsaturated)–1 teaspoon
Soy mayonnaise–1½ teaspoons

PLAN C—CANDIDIASIS

30 percent protein
45 to 50 percent yeast-free, wheat-free, low-glycemic carbohydrates
20 to 25 percent poly or monounsaturated (omega-3 rich) fat

For serving sizes, see page 203.

1,200 CALORIES PER DAY

Breakfast

1 serving grains and starches
1 serving protein

1 serving milk and dairy
1 serving fat

Snack
1 serving fruit

Lunch
1 serving vegetables
2 servings grains and starches
2 servings protein

Snack
1 serving protein or fruit

Dinner
1 serving vegetables
2 servings protein
1 serving fat

Snack
1 serving protein or fruit

Total: 16 servings

1,500 CALORIES PER DAY

Breakfast
1 serving grains and starches
2 servings protein
1 serving milk and dairy
1 serving fat

Snack
1 serving fruit

Lunch
1 serving vegetables
2 servings grains and starches

2 servings protein
1 serving fat

Snack

1 serving protein or fruit

Dinner

2 servings vegetables
2 servings protein
1 serving grains and starches
1 serving fat

Snack

1 serving protein or fruit

Total: 20 servings

1,800 CALORIES PER DAY

Breakfast

2 servings grains and starches
3 servings protein
1 serving milk and dairy
1 serving fat

Snack

1 serving fruit

Lunch

2 servings vegetables
2 servings grains and starches
2 servings protein
1 serving fat

Snack

1 serving protein or fruit

Dinner
2 servings vegetables
2 servings protein
2 servings grains and starches
1 serving fat

Snack
1 serving protein or fruit

Total: 24 servings

2,100 CALORIES PER DAY

Breakfast
1 serving fruit
2 servings grains and starches
2 servings protein
1 serving milk and dairy
1 serving fat

Snack
1 serving fruit

Lunch
3 servings vegetables
2 servings grains and starches
3 servings protein
1 serving fat

Snack
1 serving protein or fruit

Dinner
3 servings vegetables
3 servings protein
2 servings grains and starches
1 serving fat

Snack
1 serving protein or fruit

Total: 28 servings

FOODS TO AVOID

- Foods high in sugar (brown, granulated, maple, date, turbinado, powdered), dextrose, fructose, galactose, glucose, glycogen, lactose (milk sugar), maltose, mannitol, monosaccharides, polysaccharides, sorbitol, sucrose, and molasses
- Artificial sweeteners, including NutraSweet, Equal, and saccharin (Stevia natural extract can be used in moderation)
- Table salt
- Milk products
- Caffeine
- Foods containing citric acid
- Yeast and yeasted products, including alcoholic beverages (beer, champagne, liquors, wine), bread, and pastry
- Mushrooms, cheeses with rinds, coffee, most teas, condiments containing vinegar (ketchup, mustard, mayonnaise, salad dressing), fermented foods and drinks (cider, root beer), bottled or canned fruit juices, dried fruits, strawberries, melons, canned fruits, leftovers (older than twenty-four hours), malted products (barley malt, malted milk, cereals, candies), peanuts, pistachios, peanut oil, peanut butter, processed and/or smoked meats and fish (beef jerky, corned beef, hot dogs, luncheon meats, pastrami, sausages), pickled foods, tempeh, and miso

SERVING SIZES

Fruit
Fruit must always be fresh and juice should preferably be fresh squeezed.

Apple–1 small
Berries–1 cup
Cherries–10 large
Grapefruit–½ small

Grapes–½ cup
Orange–1 small
Peach–1 medium
Plums–2 medium
Watermelon–1 cup

Vegetables

Starred vegetables (*): One serving equals ½ cup.
Unstarred vegetables: Use as desired.

Alfalfa sprouts
Artichokes
Asparagus
Broccoli
Brussels sprouts
Cabbage
Cauliflower
Celery
Chickpeas*
Cucumbers
Dark green leafy vegetables (chard, spinach)
Eggplant
Green beans
Green peas*
Green peppers
Okra
Onions*
Parsnips*
Pumpkin*
Radishes
Red peppers
Rutabagas*
Salad vegetables (chicory, endive, lettuce, parsley, watercress)
Spinach
String beans
Summer squash
Tomatoes
Turnips*
Vegetable juice*

Wax beans
Winter squash*
Zucchini*

Grains and Starches

Spelt bread–½ slice
Rice and Shine cereal–¾ cup
Quinoa, cooked–¾ cup
Brown rice, cooked–½ cup
Popcorn, popped (no butter)–1 cup
Corn polenta, cooked–⅓ cup
Yeast-free bread–½ slice
Tinkyada, 100% rice pasta, cooked–⅔ cup
Van's yeast-free, gluten-free waffles–1

Protein

Baked beans–½ cup
Cheese (American)–2-ounce slice
Egg**–1 medium
Egg beaters or egg whites**–¼ cup
Lentils–1 cup
Red meat (beef, free-range)*–2 ounces
Sesame seeds–1½ tablespoons
Sunflower seeds–1½ tablespoons
Sea bass–2 ounces
Cod–3 ounces
Haddock–3 ounces
Halibut–3 ounces
Lobster**–1 ounce
Mackerel–3 ounces
Salmon–3 ounces
Scallops–2 ounces
Shrimp–2 ounces
Red snapper–3 ounces
Swordfish–2 ounces
Trout–2 ounces
Tuna (steak)–1 ounce
Tuna, canned (water packed)–1 ounce
Chicken (white meat, skinless, free-range)–2 ounces

Exhibit 6.1 Weekly Food Log

Week _____

	Day 1		Day 2		Day 3		Day 4		Day 5		Day 6		Day 7	
	SV	Food	SV	Food	SV	Food	SV	Food	SV	Food	SV	Food	SV	Food
Breakfast														
Snack														
Lunch														
Snack														
Dinner														
Snack														

Turkey (white meat, skinless, free-range)–2 ounces
100% protein powder–⅓ ounce

* Limit to once a week (leanest cut).
** Allowed if you're not allergic.

Milk and Dairy

Rice Dream–½ cup
Cheese (American)–2-ounce slice
Lactaid (lactose-free milk)–1 cup

Fat

Almond butter–⅓ teaspoon
Almonds–4 medium
Avocado–⅛ medium
Canola oil–½ teaspoon
Guacamole–1 tablespoon
Olive oil–¾ teaspoon
Olives–5 small
Margarine (polyunsaturated)–1 teaspoon

CHAPTER SEVEN

ENERGY BLOCK ACUTHERAPY

It's one of the most common mistakes to
consider that the limit of our power of perception
is also the limit of all there is to perceive.

C. W. LEADBEATER

One day I found a videotape on my desk that was sent by a friend. I tossed it into a drawer, where it got lost in a sea of junk. It was about two years later when my wife discovered the tape. Something about it intrigued her, so she decided to give it a watch. Next thing you know, I was watching it, too, and couldn't believe my eyes. Some guy, by "tapping" on people and having them focus on things they feared, was helping them overcome phobias, such as a fear of heights or snakes.

A few days later, while I was telling a client about the tape, it occurred to me that it might be fun to test this technique on her. First, I asked if she had any really bad habits or long-standing fears. She said that ever since breaking her leg while skiing when she was sixteen, she hadn't gone skiing at all for fear that she might break her leg again. Before her injury she had been skiing competitively for years.

I then asked her to rate her fear on a scale of one to ten (ten being extremely fearful and one being no fear at all). She said it was a ten and that she had never feared anything more. Next, I had her imagine herself on skis, going down a slope, and while she focused on this, I had her tap the appropriate points. After two or three minutes, I asked her again to rate her fear. "It's gone!" she replied, astonished. "Tell me, what in the world did you do?" "I'm not really sure," I said, "and to tell you the truth, I'm surprised it worked!"

When I saw her about a week later, she had some very exciting news. "Guess what?" she shouted proudly. "A few days ago, I actually skied! I had a really great time and didn't have even a twinge of fear! Whatever you did was amazing—I can't believe my fear is gone!"

It was at this point I added "energy work" to my bag of tricks. At first, I used it to help people conquer addictions, cravings, and fears, and mainly used the treatment techniques that I learned from tapes and books. Then, as I gained more confidence in my instinct and level of skill, I started to think of different ways to apply everything I had learned. Again and again, I continued to be amazed at the results. This was when I began using energy work to address UFOs.

If I hadn't seen it benefit so many people, so many times, I'd be hesitant to discuss such a "radical" concept in this book, mainly because most people are quick to assume it's New Age bunk. This is really a shame because whether people believe it or not, the fact is that this therapy, strange as it seems, can have startling results. And the way I figure it, even if you're suspicious of things like this, it's easy to do and doesn't take long, so what have you got to lose?

The pioneer of this therapy is Roger Callahan, Ph.D. (the person my wife and I observed many years ago on that tape). He calls it thought field therapy, often referred to as TFT. Variations of TFT, such as emotional freedom techniques (EFT), use similar protocols but emphasize different treatment techniques. The approach I use combines both TFT and EFT but reflects my own experience using different sequences and points. My name for it is energy block acutherapy (EBA).

For those who are unfamiliar with energy therapies, let me explain. Essentially, they are a means to reveal and eliminate *energy blocks*—blocks that hinder the energy flow in our body's energy fields. (I know—I found this hard to believe the first time I heard it, too!) Energy fields are a little hard to explain, but here's my take: In Chinese medicine, treatment involves helping people to balance their qi. Qi (pronounced "chee") is the energy our body stores or "holds" that *can*, if it is imbalanced, trigger illness, pain, and distress. Qi is also the energy of our feelings, thoughts, and beliefs, and the places, or channels, where qi exists are sometimes called *thought fields*. It's in these fields that energy blocks give birth to UFOs. So if, for example, you hold a belief in your energy field that you're weak, your body will think it must be a fact and behave like it truly is.

Energy therapies work by stimulating meridian points, the same points acupuncturists use to help their patients heal (meridians are the channels, or energy pathways, that they treat). EBA works by tapping, rubbing, and focusing on these points, as do energy therapies such as TFT and EFT. Depending on the treatment approach, affirmations may also be used, but the right exercises and sequence of "taps" is what really makes this work.

When combined with movements and sounds that stimulate different parts of the brain, EBA triggers a powerful shift in how people feel and think. This therapy can treat addictions, fears, and performance-related slumps, as well as cravings, self-sabotage, and post-traumatic stress. All of these problems could easily cause or act as UFOs—UFOs that this type of energy work can directly address.

While I've found that this therapy works amazingly fast (eight times out of ten), on occasion I find that people have blocks that require extra time to address (sometimes there are many layers that must be considered one at a time). For example, if you are treating yourself to conquer a fear of heights, a feeling or memory that you've suppressed may suddenly be revealed. Consequently, you may bring to light some unforeseen concerns.

If you think the way acupuncture is said to work is a bit far-fetched, you're apt to conclude that energy work is a fanciful concept, too. But like I said, you've got nothing to lose, so I hope you'll give it a try.

ENERGY BLOCK ACUTHERAPY (EBA)

EBA treatments are best performed in a place where you won't be disturbed (you will need to focus intently on your concern for a good result). I also suggest making copies of the treatment techniques you require and keeping them in your wallet or purse to use at appropriate times.

Before any treatment, rate how you feel on a scale of one to ten. If you feel your problem couldn't be worse, your rating should be a ten. If you feel you have no problem at all, your rating should be a one. Once you've concluded a treatment, promptly rate your problem again. If your rating is not yet a one, repeat the treatment right away, this time using the breathing exercise below before you begin. If your rating still hasn't dropped to one by the time you've completed these steps, use the multipurpose treatment sequence (page 223).

BREATHING EXERCISE

Cross your left leg over your right and your right hand over your left. Now interlace your fingers and twist your hands so they lie on your chest. Inhale very slowly, resting your tongue on the roof of your mouth. Then exhale very slowly, resting your tongue on the floor of your mouth. Repeat for two or three minutes or until you feel relaxed.

MUSCLE TEST TO DETERMINE
IF YOU'RE ENERGETICALLY REVERSED

To see if you have an energy block at the root of a UFO, ask somebody you trust to help you perform the following test:

1. Hold one arm out straight to the side and parallel to the floor.
2. Have your partner put his or her hand on your arm or on top of your wrist.
3. Imagine yourself feeling anxious about the issue you'd like to test. For example, close your eyes and imagine yourself craving something sweet. Focus intently on any negative thoughts that come to mind.
4. Now, with your arm out straight, resisting your partner's downward force, say out loud, "I would like to stop craving sweets" (or whatever you crave). Your partner should note the level of strength you have when you try to resist.
5. Now repeat the procedure (using the same arm, in the same way), but this time while saying something like, "I want to keep craving sweets." If while you are making this statement you are resisting with greater strength, you may be inclined energetically to crave sweets, i.e., "reversed." If this is the case, affirmations should precede your first series of "taps."
6. The following treatments will help to release or "reprogram" energy blocks. After each treatment, use the one-to-ten scale to assess your success.

TREATMENT SEQUENCES

NEGATIVITY

While tapping the side of your hand below your knuckle (see point 16 in Figure 7.1), repeat the following statement (say it out loud or to yourself): "I accept myself unconditionally even though I (fill in the blank)." Examples of things to say are "even though I can't lose weight," or "even though I'm afraid I won't be able to get in shape." Repeat this statement *three* times while you continue to tap your hand.

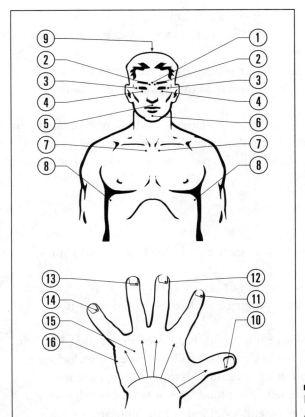

Figure 7.1
Acupoints

Now tap the following points while focused intently on your concern. (*Note:* While tapping, it helps if you say out loud what the problem is, for example, "this phobia" or "this craving I have for sweets.")

Tapping Sequence

Tap a point at least *ten* times before proceeding to the next point.

- The part of either eyebrow that is closest to your nose (2).
- The indentation about 1 inch to the side of either eye (3).
- The indentation about 1 inch directly below either eye (4).
- The uppermost part of the indentation right below your nose (5).

- The uppermost part of the indentation under your lower lip (6).
- The tender spot under your collarbone, 1 inch *below* the innermost end (7).
- Under your armpit (four finger widths) on either side of your ribs (8).
- The top of your head, in the center, in the area of your crown (9).

Now perform the following steps while tapping the back of your hand (tap point 15 firmly using a steady, rhythmic pace). Tap between the tendons on the outer top part of your hand (for this particular sequence, tap on the top of your left hand).

Bridge

- With your eyes open, look straight ahead (don't turn or lift your head).
- Close your eyes for a few seconds (again, don't turn or lift your head).
- Open your eyes (without moving your head)—look down and to the right.
- Again, without turning or lifting your head, look down and to the left.
- Whirl your eyes in a full circle (either clockwise or counterclockwise).
- Whirl your eyes in a full circle again (this time, the opposite way).
- Hum any song to yourself or out loud (one or two lines will suffice).
- Count to five very slowly (either out loud or to yourself).
- Again, hum any song (one or two lines to yourself or out loud).

Repeat the first sequence of tapping while staying focused on your concern. Then look down and slowly look up while tapping the top of your hand.

INSOMNIA AND OBSESSIVE THINKING

Breathing Exercise: Cross your left leg over your right and your right hand over your left. Now interlace your fingers and twist your hands so they lie on your chest. Inhale very slowly, resting your tongue on the roof of your mouth. Then exhale very slowly, resting your tongue on the floor of your mouth. Repeat for two or three minutes or until you feel relaxed.

While tapping the side of your hand below your knuckle (point 16), repeat the following statement (say it out loud or to yourself): "I accept myself unconditionally even though I (fill in the blank)." Examples of things to say are "even though I'm afraid I won't sleep," or "even though I'm afraid I can't escape these obsessive thoughts." Repeat this statement *three* times while you continue to tap your hand.

Now tap the following points while focused intently on your concern. (*Note:* While tapping, it helps if you say out loud what the problem is, for example, "insomnia" or "these obsessive, worrisome thoughts.")

Tapping Sequence

For the following finger and thumb points, you must tap on your left hand. Tap each point at least ten times before you tap anywhere else.

- The part of either eyebrow that is closest to your nose (2).
- The indentation about 1 inch to the side of either eye (3).
- The indentation about 1 inch directly below either eye (4).
- Under your armpit (four finger widths) on either side of your ribs (8).
- The tender spot under your collarbone, 1 inch *below* the innermost end (7).
- The cuticle of your thumbnail (lower right side of the nail) (10).
- Under your armpit (four finger widths) on either side of your ribs (8).
- The tender spot under your collarbone, 1 inch *below* the innermost end (7).
- The cuticle of your little finger (lower right side of the nail) (14).
- The tender spot under your collarbone, 1 inch *below* the innermost end (7).
- The cuticle of your index finger (lower right side of the nail) (11).
- The top of your head, in the center, in the area of your crown (9).

Now perform the following steps while tapping the back of your hand (tap point 15 firmly using a steady, rhythmic pace). Tap between the tendons on the outer top part of your hand (for this particular sequence, tap on the top of your left hand).

Bridge

- With your eyes open, look straight ahead (don't turn or lift your head).

- Close your eyes for a few seconds (again, don't turn or lift your head).
- Open your eyes (without moving your head)—look down and to the right.
- Again, without turning or lifting your head, look down and to the left.
- Whirl your eyes in a full circle (either clockwise or counterclockwise)
- Whirl your eyes in a full circle again (this time, the opposite way).
- Hum any song to yourself or out loud (one or two lines will suffice).
- Count to five very slowly (either out loud or to yourself).
- Again, hum any song (one or two lines to yourself or out loud).

Repeat the first sequence of tapping while staying focused on your concern. Then look down and slowly look up while tapping the top of your hand.

STRESS-RELATED EATING

While tapping the side of your hand below your knuckle (point 16), repeat the following statement (say it out loud or to yourself): "I accept myself unconditionally even though I (fill in the blank)." Examples of things to say are "even though stress makes me overeat," or "even though I often binge when I'm anxious, tense, or scared." Repeat this statement *three* times while you continue to tap your hand.

Now tap the following points while focused intently on your concern (*Note:* While tapping, it helps if you say out loud what the problem is, for example, "this anxiety" or "this craving I have for sweets.")

Tapping Sequence

Tap each point at least *ten* times before you tap anywhere else. For the following finger and thumb points, you must tap on your left hand.

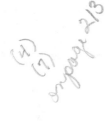

- The indentation about 1 inch directly below either eye (4).
- The tender spot under your collarbone, 1 inch *below* the innermost end (7).
- Under your armpit (four finger widths) on either side of your ribs (8).
- The cuticle of your little finger (lower right side of the nail) (14).
- The top of your head, in the center, in the area of your crown (9).

Repeat the first sequence of tapping while staying focused on your concern. Then look down and slowly look up while tapping the top of your hand.

CRAVINGS AND ADDICTIVE URGES

While tapping the side of your hand below your knuckle (point 16), repeat any one of the following statements (or create your own):

Examples of Affirmations

- "I accept myself unconditionally, even though I crave _____."
- "I accept myself unconditionally, even though I'm addicted to _____."
- "I accept myself unconditionally, even though I'm out of control."

Repeat your statement *three* times while you continue to tap your hand.

Tapping Sequence

Tap each point at least *ten* times before you tap anywhere else.

- The part of either eyebrow that is closest to your nose (2).
- The indentation about 1 inch directly below either eye (4).
- The uppermost part of the indentation right below your nose (5).
- The uppermost part of the indentation under your lower lip (6).
- Under your armpit (four finger widths) on either side of your ribs (8).
- The tender spot under your collarbone, 1 inch *below* the innermost end (7).
- The top of your head, in the center, in the area of your crown (9).
- The indentations about 1 inch directly below *both* eyes (4).

Bridge

Repeat the first sequence of tapping while staying focused on your concern. Then look down and slowly look up while tapping the back of your hand.

GENERAL ANXIETY, WORRY, AND STRESS

While tapping the side of your hand below your knuckle (point 16), repeat any one of the following statements (or create your own):

Examples of Affirmations

- "I accept myself unconditionally, even though I feel _____ ."
- "I accept myself unconditionally, and I fully release my fear."
- "I accept myself unconditionally, even though I'm afraid that I'll fail."
- "Now and forever, I fully release the deepest cause of my fear."

Repeat your statement *three* times while you continue to tap your hand.

Tapping Sequence

Tap each point at least *ten* times before you tap anywhere else.

- The indentation about 1 inch directly below either eye (4).
- The uppermost part of the indentation right below your nose (5).
- The uppermost part of the indentation under your lower lip (6).
- Under your armpit (four finger widths) on either side of your ribs (8).
- The tender spot under your collarbone, 1 inch *below* the innermost end (7).
- The top of your head, in the center, in the area of your crown (9).

Bridge

Repeat the first sequence of tapping while staying focused on your concern. Then look down and slowly look up while tapping the back of your hand.

FATIGUE

While tapping the side of your hand below your knuckle (point 16), repeat any one of the following statements (or create your own):

Examples of Affirmations

- "I accept myself unconditionally, even though I am often fatigued."
- "I accept myself unconditionally, even though I feel lazy and weak."
- "I accept myself unconditionally, even though I'm too tired to work out."
- "Now and forever, I fully release the deepest cause of my fatigue."

Repeat your statement *three* times while you continue to tap your hand.

Tapping Sequence

Tap each point at least *ten* times before you tap anywhere else.

- The part of either eyebrow that is closest to your nose (2).
- The indentation about 1 inch directly below either eye (4).
- The tender spot under your collarbone, 1 inch *below* the innermost end (7).
- The spot between the tendons on the outer top part of your hand (15).
- The top of your head, in the center, in the area of your crown (9).

Bridge

Repeat the first sequence of tapping while staying focused on your concern. Then look down and slowly look up while tapping the back of your hand.

PREMENSTRUAL SYNDROME (PMS)

While tapping the side of your hand below your knuckle (point 16), repeat any one of the following statements (or create your own):

Examples of Affirmations

- "I accept myself unconditionally, even though I feel _____."
- "I accept myself unconditionally, even though I feel out of control."
- "I accept myself unconditionally, even though I crave _____."

- "I accept myself unconditionally, even though I'm too stressed to work out."
- "Now and forever, I fully release the deepest cause of my stress."

Repeat your statement *three* times while you continue to tap your hand.

Tapping Sequence

For the following finger and thumb points, you must tap on your left hand. Tap each point at least *ten* times before you tap anywhere else.

- The top of your head, in the center, in the area of your crown (9).
- The part of either eyebrow that is closest to your nose (2).
- The uppermost part of the indentation under your lower lip (6).
- The indentation about 1 inch directly below either eye (4).
- Under your armpit (four finger widths) on either side of your ribs (8).
- The tender spot under your collarbone, 1 inch *below* the innermost end (7).
- The indentation about 1 inch directly below either eye (4).
- The cuticle of your little finger (lower right side of the nail) (14).
- The tender spot under your collarbone, 1 inch *below* the innermost end (7).
- The top of your head, in the center, in the area of your crown (9).

Bridge

Repeat the first sequence of tapping while staying focused on your concern. Then look down and slowly look up while tapping the back of your hand.

PROCRASTINATION

While tapping the side of your hand below your knuckle (point 16), repeat any one of the following statements (or create your own):

Examples of Affirmations

- "I accept myself unconditionally, even though I've been putting things off."

- "I accept myself unconditionally, even if I *keep* putting things off."
- "I accept myself unconditionally, even though I've put off working out."
- "Now and forever, I fully release the deepest cause of this block."

Repeat your statement *three* times while you continue to tap your hand.

Tapping Sequence

For the following finger and thumb points, you must tap on your left hand. Tap each point at least *ten* times before you tap anywhere else.

- Directly between your eyebrows (tap with three fingers or your palm) (1).
- The part of either eyebrow that is closest to your nose (2).
- The uppermost part of the indentation right below your nose (5).
- The uppermost part of the indentation under your lower lip (6).
- The indentation about 1 inch directly below either eye (4).
- The tender spot under your collarbone, 1 inch *below* the innermost end (7).
- Under your armpit (four finger widths) on either side of your ribs (8).
- The tender spot under your collarbone, 1 inch *below* the innermost end (7).
- The indentation about 1 inch directly below either eye (4).
- The top of your head, in the center, in the area of your crown (9).

Bridge

Repeat the first sequence of tapping while staying focused on your concern. Then look down and slowly look up while tapping the back of your hand.

EMOTIONAL TRAUMA

Breathing Exercise: Cross your left leg over your right and your right hand over your left. Now interlace your fingers and twist your hands so they lie on your chest. Inhale very slowly, resting your tongue on the roof of your mouth. Then exhale very slowly, resting your tongue on the floor of your mouth. Repeat for two or three minutes or until you feel relaxed.

While tapping the side of your hand below your knuckle (point 16), repeat any one of the following statements (or create your own):

Examples of Affirmations

- "I accept myself unconditionally, even though I feel fragile and weak."
- "I accept myself unconditionally, even if I am not in control."
- "I accept myself unconditionally, even though I don't always feel safe."
- "Now and forever, I fully release the deepest cause of this fear."

Repeat your statement *three* times while you continue to tap your hand.

Tapping Sequence

For the following finger and thumb points, you must tap on your left hand. Tap each point at least *ten* times before you tap anywhere else.

- Directly between your eyebrows (tap with three fingers or your palm) (1).
- The part of either eyebrow that is closest to your nose (2).
- The indentation about 1 inch to the side of either eye (3).
- Under your armpit (four finger widths) on either side of your ribs (8).
- The tender spot under your collarbone, 1 inch *below* the innermost end (7).
- The cuticle of your thumbnail (lower right side of the nail) (10).
- The tender spot under your collarbone, 1 inch *below* the innermost end (7).
- The cuticle of your index finger (lower right side of the nail) (11).
- The tender spot under your collarbone, 1 inch *below* the innermost end (7).
- The cuticle of your little finger (lower right side of the nail) (14).
- The tender spot under your collarbone, 1 inch *below* the innermost end (7).
- Under your armpit (four finger widths) on either side of your ribs (8).
- The top of your head, in the center, in the area of your crown (9).

Bridge

Repeat the first sequence of tapping while staying focused on your concern. Then look down and slowly look up while tapping the back of your hand.

GENERAL PHOBIAS

While tapping the side of your hand below your knuckle (point 16), repeat any one of the following statements (or create your own):

Examples of Affirmations

- "I accept myself unconditionally, even though I'm afraid of _____."
- "I accept myself unconditionally, even though I feel trapped by my fear."
- "Now and forever, I fully release the deepest cause of this fear."

Repeat your statement *three* times while you continue to tap your hand.

Tapping Sequence

Tap each point at least *ten* times before you tap anywhere else.

- The part of either eyebrow that is closest to your nose (2).
- The uppermost part of the indentation right below your nose (5).
- The indentation about 1 inch directly below either eye (4).
- Under your armpit (four finger widths) on either side of your ribs (8).
- The tender spot under your collarbone, 1 inch *below* the innermost end (7).
- The top of your head, in the center, in the area of your crown (9).

Bridge

Repeat the first sequence of tapping while staying focused on your concern. Then look down and slowly look up while tapping the back of your hand.

MULTIPURPOSE SEQUENCE

Use this sequence for *any* concern (or when other treatments fail).

Breathing Exercise: Cross your left leg over your right and your right hand over your left. Now interlace your fingers and twist your hands so they lie on your chest. Inhale very slowly, resting your tongue on the roof of your mouth. Then exhale very slowly, resting your tongue on the floor of your mouth. Repeat for two or three minutes or until you feel relaxed.

While tapping the side of your hand below your knuckle (point 16), repeat any one of the following statements (or create your own):

Examples of Affirmations

- "I accept myself unconditionally, even though I'm afraid of _____."
- "I accept myself unconditionally, even if I _____."
- "Now and forever, I fully release the deepest cause of this _____."

Repeat your statement *three* times while you continue to tap your hand.

Tapping Sequence

For the following finger and thumb points, you must tap on your left hand. Tap each point at least *ten* times before you tap anywhere else.

- The part of either eyebrow that is closest to your nose (2).
- The indentation about 1 inch to the side of either eye (3).
- The indentation about 1 inch directly below either eye (4).
- The uppermost part of the indentation right below your nose (5).
- The uppermost part of the indentation under your lower lip (6).
- The tender spot under your collarbone, 1 inch *below* the innermost end (7).
- Under your armpit (four finger widths) on either side of your ribs (8).
- The cuticle of your index finger (lower right side of the nail) (11).
- The tender spot under your collarbone, 1 inch *below* the innermost end (7).
- The cuticle of your middle finger (lower right side of the nail) (12).
- The tender spot under your collarbone, 1 inch *below* the innermost end (7).
- The top of your head, in the center, in the area of your crown (9).

Bridge

Repeat the first sequence of tapping while staying focused on your concern. Then look down and slowly look up while tapping the back of your hand.

PART TWO

The Makeovers

Change is not something you do.
It's something you allow.
       Will Garcia

At first, when publishers gave me feedback about my idea for this book, most were concerned that doing a project like this was too much of a risk. The risk, they said, was not being sure how the makeovers would turn out. To me, though, this was a *good* thing—it would ensure that the stories were *real*. I say this because the pictures we usually see show uncommon results, and the stories we hear, while inspiring, make many of us set impractical goals. Moreover, too often the stories are trite, embellished, or hard to believe. We rarely hear about what went *wrong* or the things that could get in our way.

So instead of just telling the stories of those who had problem-free, best-case results, I chose seven people at random, taking the "risk" that some wouldn't succeed (as opposed to choosing only the best of thousands who followed the plan). What happened to these seven people could very easily happen to you. They stumbled, fell down, and got up—many times—but transformed themselves as a result.

I am grateful to all of these people for being so willing to tell the truth. They were all a pleasure to work with and experienced great success. I'm honored to share their stories and trust they will offer you strength and hope. If nothing else, you will see how to make stepping-stones out of stumbling blocks.

CHAPTER EIGHT

CLAUDIA

If you have made mistakes . . . there is always another chance for you.
You may have a fresh start any moment you choose, for this thing we
call "failure" is not the falling down, but the staying down.

MARY PICKFORD

Claudia

Age: 45
Height: 5'6"
Weight: 157 lbs.
Occupation: Curriculum Specialist *Everyday Mathematics* (SRA McGraw-Hill)

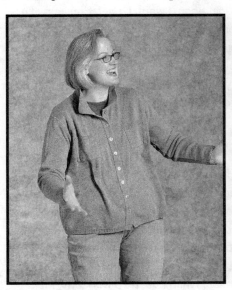 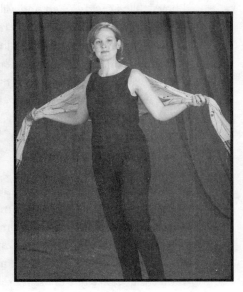

Excerpt from letter:

I was thin until I turned thirty, then I gradually let myself go. It's hard
for me to accept that I have to work now to be healthy and fit. And I'm
often confused by conflicting advice—I don't know what to believe!

Journal Entry #1

Hi Michael,

Thank you for this opportunity! It really is quite exciting!

Being observed during this process will be a new experience for me. My initial impression is that it will be both a good thing and a bad thing. Good, because I'll be getting support and advice from experts, and I won't want to let anyone down—especially myself! Bad, because I'll have to be very honest to derive the most benefit from this project. Which means that I'll have to come to terms with everything I've been denying about my situation. What I discover may not be pretty. But you know, as I get older I find there is a lot of freedom in being honest about who I am and how I feel. Okay, so maybe it won't be so bad after all! (Please forgive my circuitous thinking!)

Journal Entry #2

Hi Michael,

I have called Gold's Gym and will join soon. I want to get familiar with the layout before we start (to remove the intimidation factor).

I don't know why, but I have an image of Gold's as being a place for the "body beautiful." I hope I'll feel comfortable there and that my preconceived notions are all in my head (actually, isn't everything?). Don't worry—I won't get buff before you take the "before" shots!

Journal Entry #3

Michael has asked me to keep a food log. I think knowing that I have to write everything down will make me think twice before eating something that isn't good for me. Another case of good/bad. For the time being, it will make me more aware, but for the long run, what will I do when I'm the only one watching? I don't *think* my diet is bad. But to be honest, I don't think about it a lot. I think more about the fact that I don't get enough exercise. When I used to work out, I felt like it cut a huge hole in my day. And it felt tedious—like a task—even on days when I had a good workout! I wonder if it's because for most of my life I've been fit without having to work at it. Now that I read what I just wrote, I realize that when I say most of my life it really isn't true. Maybe half of my life, and as time goes on, maybe less than half!

I started becoming aware of my body changing (for the worse) after I had my second child. Noah is going to be 18 in January! This is a long time to feel out of control. I hope I can live with the changes I'll have to make. My job requires me to be home on the phone, at the computer, or traveling. Home is fine because I have choices and can prepare my own food. But I'm sitting way too much! When I travel, I have less choice about what (and when) I eat, and except for when I'm presenting, I'm sitting a lot as well.

Week 1—Journal Entry #4

Hi Michael,
Well, I joined the gym today and spent most of the afternoon there. The people at the gym were very nice, but it was all so overwhelming! Too many machines, too much to remember! I wasn't even sure that I was on the right piece of equipment—let alone if I was using it properly. HELP!

I tried to remember the exercises that you showed me, but some of them were running together in my mind. I spent a lot of time

---

CLAUDIA

Weight, girth measurements, and body fat percentage, before:

Height: 5'6"
Weight: 157 lbs.
Chest (bust): 35"
Waist: 30½"
Hips: 43"
Upper thighs: 23" (L), 22¾" (R)
Calves: 14⅝" (L), 14¾" (R)
Ankles: 9" (L), 9" (R)
Upper arms: 12½" (L), 12½" (R)
Forearms: 9⅞" (L), 10" (R)
Wrists: 6⅛" (L), 6⅛" (R)
Body fat: 31%

---

wandering aimlessly around the gym, looking for machines that might fit the description of the ones you suggested. I am sure that everyone thought I'd lost my marbles!

I'm hoping that you'll straighten me out once we meet at Gold's. I'm looking forward to it!

Reply from Michael

Hi Claudia,

Not to worry! Almost everyone has a similar experience on their first visit to the gym. All of the stuff that seems so complicated and intimidating now will seem very simple in only a few days or weeks. I promise!

Regarding your UFO test—let's deal with your top three issues first. Then, once we do, we'll assess where you stand and see what is left to address.

It looks like we need to start you on Plan C (for candidiasis) and get you a full-spectrum, bright-light source (for SAD). We'll discuss any issues that come up around perfectionism as needed. With regard to a DHEA imbalance and/or food intolerances—let's see what happens once we cut out the yeast. If after three or four weeks you're still experiencing symptoms, we'll address these problems then.

Question: Do you think the energy work we did to address your anxiety about the photo shoot was helpful? You seemed very much at ease!

See you soon!

CLAUDIA'S UFOs

Candidiasis
Perfectionism
Seasonal Affective Disorder (SAD)
DHEA Imbalance
Body Dysmorphic Disorder (BDD)
Attention Deficit Disorder (ADD)
Seasonal Allergies
"Askaphobia" (Fear of Asking for Help)
Food Intolerances
Insufficient Exercise Intensity

Hi Michael,
Yes, with regard to the photo session, I think the tapping (energy work) you did with me really helped.

And yes, I would prefer eggs to red meat, so let me know what that means for amounts. Also, for breakfast, are these all the protein choices I have? I see cheese, eggs, lentils, and beans. But the rest is meat and fish (I think these foods would be hard to stomach first thing in the morning). What do you recommend?

Reply from Michael

Hi Claudia,
One medium egg equals one serving. Other protein options (for breakfast): protein powder and/or fruit mixed with juice, water, or milk. Just make sure the powder has no (or very little) sugar and doesn't contain any gluten or yeast (in keeping with Plan C).

Week 2—Journal Entry #6

Hi Michael,
I'm feeling stronger! It's a good feeling! I feel much better now that you showed me the ropes.

Foodwise, it's a bit of a different story. I'm feeling somewhat deprived—not hungry, just not satisfied.

Believe it or not, I actually bought some new clothes! Everything seems to fit better already! Only tops, though. I'm not sure I want to invest in skirts or pants yet—I'm planning on dropping a size or so—Have a good week, I'll write when I return . . .

Week 3—Journal Entry #7

Hi Michael,
Random thoughts:

Regarding Resistance Training and the Gym
I was incredibly frustrated the first time I visited Gold's. I probably tried to accomplish too much in one visit. Getting used to a new

gym and trying to figure out the layout was a challenge. I'm still uncomfortable with the "maleness" of this facility.

I like the series of resistance exercises that you gave me, and I love the stretches—something I've never spent much time doing before. They make me feel more limber and "safe." When I do them, I don't feel like I'm going to hurt myself (when I use the equipment).

This program has produced results very quickly. I already feel *much* stronger and, surprisingly, determined to keep this up. Most of the exercises are easy to do correctly. A few, like the abdominal and back exercises, still don't feel quite right to me. I may need to work on my technique.

I'm disappointed that on my last business trip I didn't have a chance to work out. I had every intention to, but it wasn't to be. I can't blame my schedule or a lack of opportunity. I was exhausted and had some work to finish. This was enough to override my intention to go to the gym. But I did get as far as putting my sweats and shoes on!

> " This program has produced results very quickly. I already feel *much* stronger and, surprisingly, determined to keep this up. "

Cardiovascular Exercise

I want to improve my efforts in this area. I think it will be the key to seeing significant fat loss (along with the anticandida diet). I have been walking and using the elliptical trainer, but I am so bored with these things that I feel like I'm going through the motions.

Light Box

Today I am ordering a bright-light source for my office and bulbs for the lamp next to my bed (where I read a lot). I look forward to seeing if they help. This year seems better than others (with regard to SAD). Maybe it's because I've been traveling so much (getting out of my house and office).

Goals and Dreams

Right now I could use more time to do things I enjoy, for example, traveling, taking a class (for pleasure), and entertaining. I've read and followed the advice in a book called *LifeWorkTransitions.Com*. Many of the ideas in it helped me move from teaching children in a school to being an educator in a business environment.

Claudia

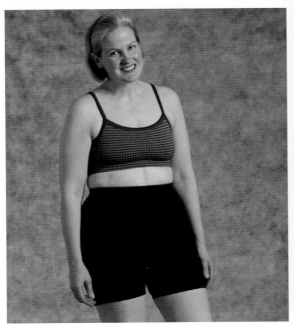

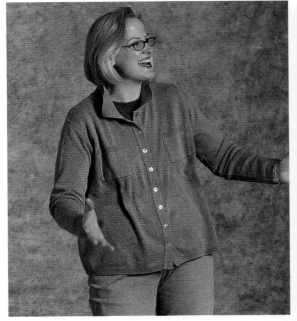

Before

After

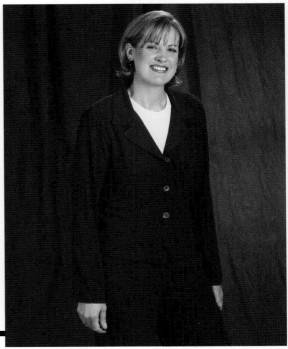

Bob

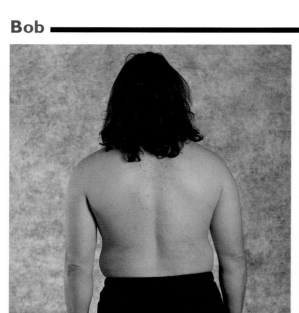

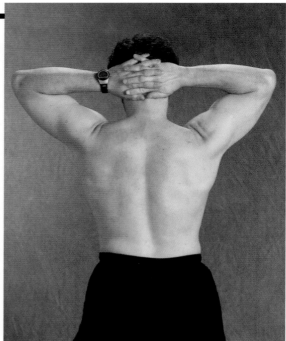

Before

After

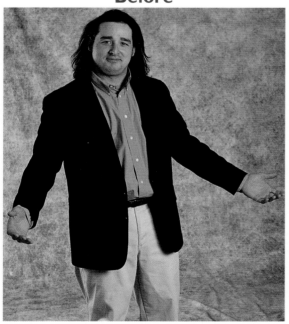

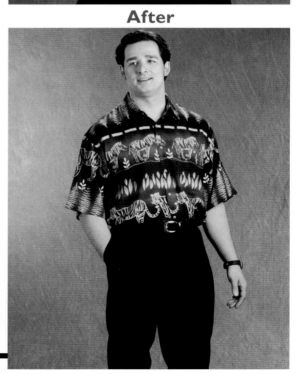

Chet

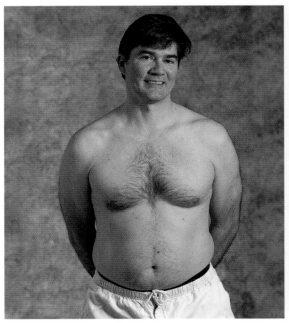

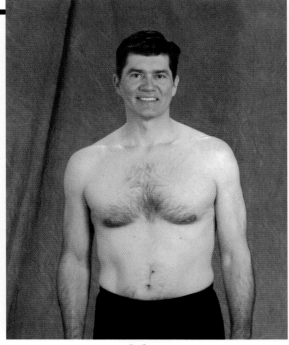

Before

After

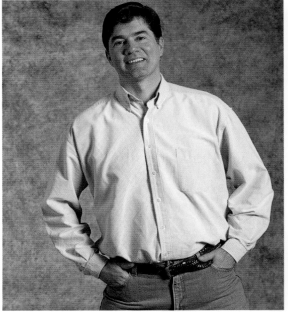

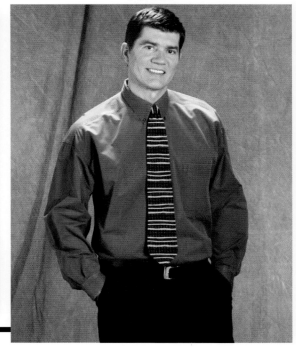

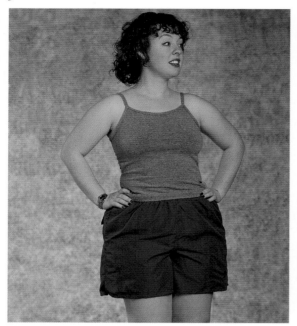

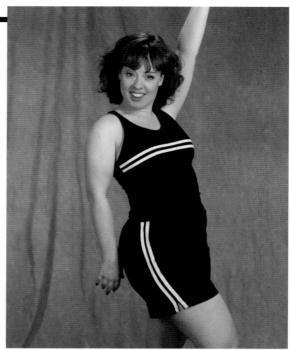

Before

After

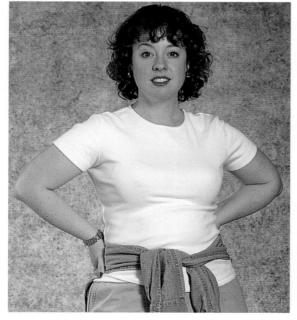

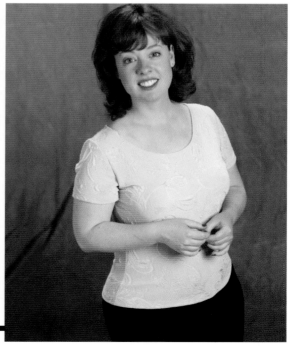

L'Tanya

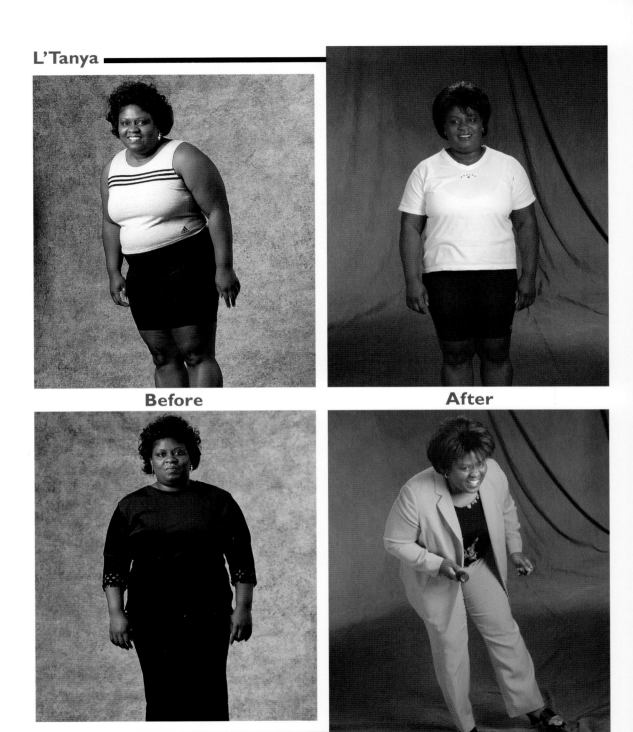

Before

After

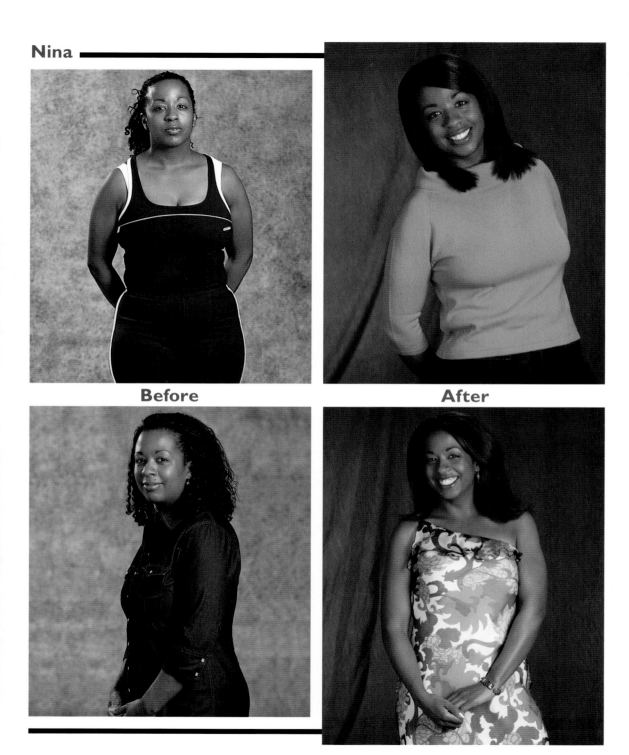

Nina

Before

After

Mandy

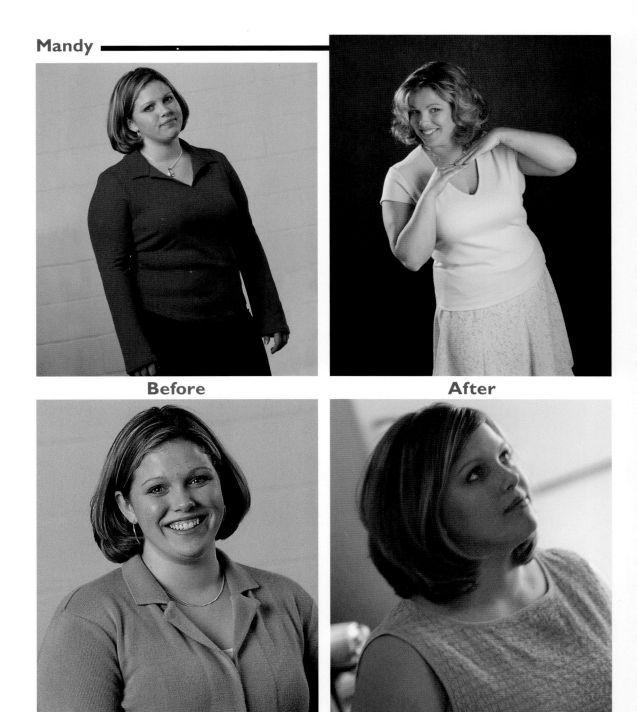

Before

After

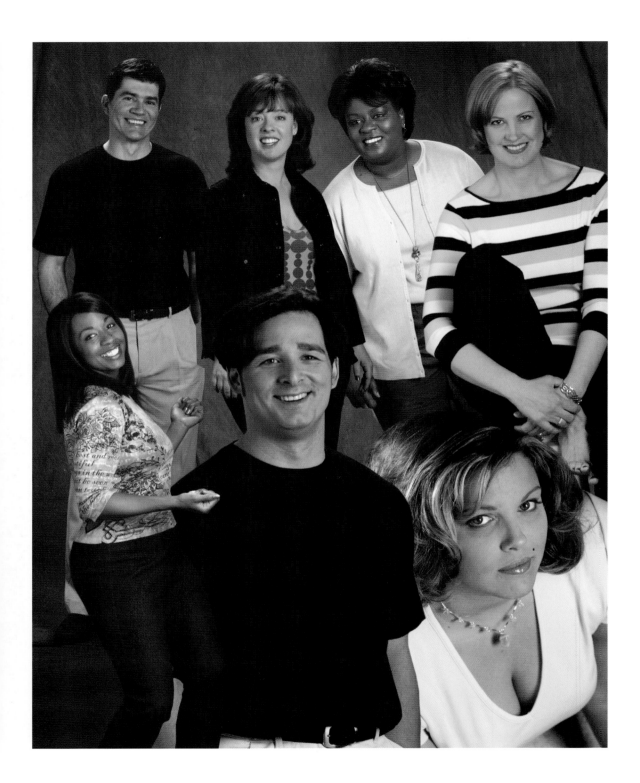

Diet

This is a source of frustration. I am working very hard to be "good" (probably sticking to 80 to 85 percent of the plan). But I think the yeast-free cookbooks I've looked at are either too restrictive or not restrictive enough (no sugar, yeast, wheat flour, alcohol, dairy, or eggs vs. pretty close to the plan I'm on). I'm not sure if my priority is reducing calories, addressing my problem with candida, or improving my general health. I'm a little confused because there are foods allowed on my plan that aren't allowed on others, for example, eggs, cheese, and fruit.

I'll admit that when I'm good about avoiding bread, pasta, pastry, sugar, and alcohol, it makes a significant difference. I feel less sluggish and have lots more energy, and the loss of weight (or the feeling that I have lost weight) is wonderful! What I miss most, though, is my glass of wine in the evening and an occasional piece of bread. I have not tried alternative (yeast- and wheat-free) pasta yet. Maybe it will help me to feel less deprived. I guess what I really want to know, or understand, is how this diet (or future diets) will play out. I know that I will not spend the rest of my life on such a restrictive plan! I think I can live without sweets (surprisingly, they have been the easiest to do without). And as far as alcohol goes, I have little desire for beer or liquor, but I really enjoy a glass of wine every now and then. Sometimes I think it's the strictness (of the candida plan) that makes the need (for wine and bread) seem greater than the actual desire. I didn't drink wine every night before starting this diet, but now that I can't have it at all, I feel deprived (mentally).

Reply from Michael

Hi Claudia,
You can eat a little cheese every now and then, as long as it's not a type with a rind. And eggs are fine (unless you're allergic).

Signs that the diet is working: more energy, quicker and easier weight loss, clearer thinking, better sleep, less stomach discomfort, less gas, less bloat, less anxiety, and improved mood—all of which will become more obvious over time.

Once you have three to six months under your belt, you can add some foods that are currently not allowed. Until then, just do the best you can! If you find that you continue to crave certain things, let me know (some energy work may help).

Week 4—Journal Entry #8

Hi Michael,
I am starting to feel much better about the changes you advised regarding my diet. I know that I will include some "bad" foods eventually, but I don't think that I'll want a steady diet of them (like I did before). I definitely have more energy. I also think that I'll keep up the weight training—it feels so good to me (as does the stretching). I'm also getting more used to Gold's. I'm still struggling with the cardio, though. For the most part, it's boring. I do it, but I don't look forward to it like I do lifting weights.

I went clothes shopping with my sister on Sunday afternoon. I notice that when things fit me better, my first thought is "What if my weight loss is only temporary? What if I gain it all back?" I'm hesitant to spend money buying clothes for a "temporary body." Or I think, "What if I continue to lose weight and need an even smaller size?" Go figure . . .

Week 5—Journal Entry #9

Hi Michael,
I feel like I haven't talked to you in so-o-o-o long! This past week has been incredibly busy. Talk about pressure! Wednesday and Thursday I drove all over southern New Jersey (to do five more presentations!). I was pleased that I was able to use the hotel gym on Tuesday afternoon (I did thirty minutes of cardio). It was the only opportunity that I had to exercise. My mornings started very early and by the end of the day I was exhausted (more emotionally than physically.) I got home Thursday night at 11:30 P.M. and was still paying for it Friday afternoon. I took a two-to-three hour nap (not something I usually need to do!).

I worked out at Gold's on Saturday morning. I missed more days than I expected (when I was away), but I picked right up where I left off with the resistance training. Fortunately, I'll be home (more often) for the next two weeks.

While there haven't been many people who've mentioned (or noticed) that I look any different, my husband says that I'm "wasting away!" But I think he really does like that I am leaner and in better shape. At the same time, I'm afraid that he has to be careful about what he says to me. For instance, if he likes what he sees too much, does this mean that he didn't like me the way I was? I don't envy his role in all of this. He knows that I listen carefully to everything he says!

I felt so good when I was packing last weekend. While I haven't purchased a lot of new clothes, my old ones fit much better. I don't feel the need to hide anymore under bulky jackets and sweaters. Now I can wear a belt or clingy clothes without feeling huge! My confidence has improved considerably, which was one of my primary goals when I started this project.

I've weighed myself several times the past few days and it looks like I am 145 pounds! Not bad! When we started, I think I was pushing 160. The diet still feels restrictive to me, but not nearly as much as in the beginning. What I find so interesting is that I think my head wants certain forbidden foods more than my body does. For instance, butter doesn't appeal to me anymore. It suddenly seems too "heavy." And anytime that I try anything sweet, it tastes *too* sweet. I don't find it appealing. I'm also surprised that I no longer miss eating pasta and bread. I like leaving the table full but without feeling so bloated and "stuffed." Also, these first six weeks have been *hard* work, and I'm determined not to lose what I've gained (or gain what I've lost!). It will be interesting to see what happens once the twelve weeks are up and you're no longer watching me. I really think I'm past doing this just for this project—but time will tell.

Week 6—Journal Entry #10

Dear "Dr. Evil,"
I just got back from the gym! The Cycle 4 routine was not as overwhelming as it felt the first time. Also, the new calf exercise you showed me is great—I can really feel it! And I love my new weight lifting gloves (even though I think I look like a geek!).

I also wanted to thank you for your last E-mail (Monday). It was nice to get an update on how everyone is doing. And you said such wonderful, encouraging things—thank you!

I continue to think about how I'll do once the project is over. I know that I'll be successful (yes, I *do* believe that!), but I want to realign my thinking so that it "fits" the new, healthier me. Right now, I'm concerned that my fear (of gaining the weight back) is the only thing that will keep me on track. Maybe my fear of losing all the ground I've gained is not a bad thing, but it isn't the way I want to be thinking. I want to be looking forward to having more success! This, as opposed to looking back and fearing what could go wrong.

Having my clothes fit better is such a nice feeling. I don't know if I'm a whole size smaller yet, but everything I wear seems to be looser and more comfortable.

Lately I've been realizing that I would like more opportunities to express my creativity. I have no artistic outlet. I would love to take a class, pick up my sketch pad, rejoin the chorus, take dancing lessons with my husband, and even learn how to play golf! But these things are so far down on my list of priorities that I fear they will never see the light of day. I think that part of the reason for this is my fear of failure, i.e., being judged on my abilities (or inabilities). I have vivid memories of the criticism I received when I was a young girl trying to play the piano, sing, draw, or dance (ballet). I don't remember getting much encouragement.

Week 7—Journal Entry #11

Hi Michael,
This past week has been a little frustrating. I can't seem to get below 143–144 pounds. I feel like if I could break the 140 barrier the rest (5 to 10 pounds?) would be easy.

I'll be on the road for work (and a little pleasure) starting next Monday. I won't be returning until the following Tuesday night. Getting some cardiovascular exercise won't be a problem, but I'm worried that I won't be able to lift weights. I find the routine both demanding and rewarding. I can really see the results and doing it gives me the satisfaction of a job well done.

I thought you might like to know that I was at the gym the other day and a man stopped to comment on my technique. He was very complimentary. Like you predicted, I now feel that the gym is a much less intimidating place. I feel like I now know more than most people do about how to exercise properly, so I no longer feel like the "imposter" or "newcomer" that I imagined I was when I started. The fact that I am making progress (and gaining confidence!) makes the gym a much less threatening place.

Hi Michael,

You know, when I was working out the other day I said something to you that was truly profound (for me). You said that I should be proud of my success and I, of course, made one of my typical self-denigrating remarks. But then I said, "I am enjoying my success—but in a very quiet way." It's true—I don't need, or want, to shout it from the rooftops. I just want to enjoy the fact that I'm in good health. It is enough, truly, to put on clothes and not crush my spirit in tiny measures by hating the way something looks or fits. It is enough to know that a curve or a muscle is the result of hard work and determination—even if no else knows or sees it. The true power of being strong is *feeling* strong.

I sat at the pool today (85 and sunny). Around me were people of many different shapes, sizes, and ages. I saw myself in so many of the women (and girls) I observed. I watched teens taking for granted their flawless skin, lean legs, and flat stomachs. I watched tired new mothers with little bellies, totally focused on their children. I most admired the women of any age, any body type, any *size*, who sat by the pool in their swimsuits looking and feeling completely at ease! Cellulite and spider veins didn't keep them under wraps—all they cared about was being somewhere sunny and warm. The next leg of my journey is to learn to enjoy how I look—to stop obsessing about it and to appreciate what I've achieved. Until now, I've been making a bigger deal over the wrapping paper than over the gift! I want to take this new confidence out for a ride and see what she can do for the rest of my life.

> **"**
> The next leg of my journey is to learn to enjoy how I look— to stop obsessing about it and to appreciate what I've achieved. Until now, I've been making a bigger deal over the wrapping paper than over the gift! I want to take this new confidence out for a ride and see what she can do for the rest of my life.
> **"**

Week 11—Journal Entry #13

Hi Michael,

Here is what will probably be one of the last installments of my journal.

I miss being a part of the teleclasses. Even when I don't have much to say, they help me to feel connected. It has been comforting to know that everyone experiences setbacks and that the feelings and concerns I've had are not uncommon.

I definitely see my body changing. And in places I didn't expect,

Weight, girth measurements, and body fat percentage, after 12 weeks:

Height: 5'6"
Weight: 139 lbs. (–18 lbs.)
Chest (bust): 34¾" (–¼")
Waist: 29" (–1½")
Hips: 38½" (–4½")
Upper thighs: 21¼" (L), 20¾" (R) (–1¾", –2")
Calves: 14¼" (L), 14⅜" (R) (–⅜", – ⅜")
Ankles: 8½" (L), 8¾" (R) (–½", – ¼")
Upper arms: 11⅜" (L), 11⅜" (R) (–1⅛", –1⅛")
Forearms: 9¼" (L), 9½" (R) (–⅝", –½")
Wrists: 6" (L), 6" (R) (–⅛", –⅛")
Total inches lost: 15⅛"
Body fat: 20% (–11%)

like my shoulders and the top part of my arms. It seems like every day I notice something a little different (for the better!).

I have not been able to stay under 140 pounds. I've been as low as 138, but now I'm back to 140. I must admit, though, that I occasionally stray from the plan. For instance, sometimes I splurge and have a cookie, piece or bread, or glass of wine. I have yet to try the "tapping" sequence you suggested for cravings. I think I'm afraid it will work!

I'm a little disappointed because 135 pounds was my goal. I almost wish I hadn't attached a number to my idea of success. I think I did a good job, but not a great job. Sometimes I wish I weren't such a perfectionist.

Week 12—Journal Entry #14

Thanks to you, Michael, and the makeover team, for your guidance, encouragement, and support! This has been a wonderful experience and I feel very fortunate to have had your help.

Regarding the image part of the makeover: I really enjoyed shopping with Ginger. I didn't realize that I could wear so many new and different styles of clothes! I'm really enjoying my new look!

Barry was great to work with and did a great job on my color and cut. My husband loved everything! We went to a wedding in Atlanta two days after the photo shoot and he enjoyed seeing me looking and feeling so good. My boys have both commented that I "look younger" and if pressed will say I look good (I don't think they have much of an opinion one way or another!).

I can't say enough about how all the little things you showed me (in the gym) helped to increase my success. They made all the difference in the world. I feel like the strength and confidence I gained from the resistance training was fundamental to my success, even with the diet and the cardiovascular part of the program. Feeling strong is a new experience for me and one that I rather enjoy. I've also learned that my days of eating a lot of bread and pasta are pretty much over, and that when I crave these things, it's usually more mental than physical. The fact is that I feel *much* better when I don't eat them. All in all, I feel like I've come a long way and that I finally have "the tiger by the tail." Now I just have to hold on.

66

All in all, I feel like I've come a long way and that I finally have "the tiger by the tail." Now I just have to hold on.

99

CHAPTER NINE

CHET

When I abandoned my dream of competing in the Olympics, I put theidea of training (for anything) totally out of my mind. And I always compared myself (later) to who, and what, I once had been.

Chet

Age: 50
Height: 6'2½"
Weight: 212 lbs.
Occupation: Senior Partner, Energy Alliance Group

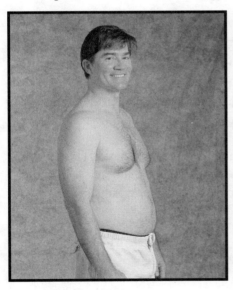 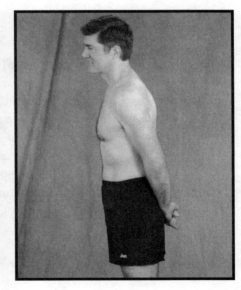

Excerpt from letter:

In college, I threw the javelin and excelled at track and field. Now I'm fifty years old and don't get much exercise at all. I also spend lots of time at work and I'm under considerable stress. But I want all of this to change . . . I want to be there for my wife and kids.

> **"**
> I'd like to return to
> who I really am
> (inside). In effect, I'd
> like to be the best
> "me" I can be.
> **"**

Journal Entry #1

Hi Michael,

Yikes! I'm on the team! This is so great . . . thank you!

Okay, some thoughts . . .

On Friday when Andrea (my wife) gave me the news, I was surprised and excited. But then I thought about the level of commitment this will require. Reality quickly set in.

Next I started thinking about the before photos. "I hope they'll be done in good taste," I said. But then I let it go. "Let them take the darn pictures," I thought. "The last ones they take are what counts!"

Another thought . . . while I'm sure that the term "makeover" is good for marketing purposes (for the book), I'm not sure it truly reflects what I hope to achieve as a result of this project. As opposed to being "made over" in a re-creation sense, I'd like to return to who I really am (inside). In effect, I'd like to be the best "me" I can be.

Well, I'm sure this is the first of many E-mails between us. I look forward to the journey!

Journal Entry #2

I was a bit stressed out today. I had a big meeting and didn't have time to prepare. It went fine, but my stress level was off the charts. Tomorrow I have another meeting. I plan to get up at 5:00 A.M.

With regard to my diet, I did pretty well today. I had a protein drink for breakfast, an apple for a mid-morning snack, a bowl of turkey chili (yes, there is such a thing!) for lunch, an orange on the way home from work, and baked haddock (with spinach) for dinner. But then it was time for dessert. I polished off two slices of pumpkin pie!

Exercise—nada. Typical day. Looking forward to the official start of my program!

Journal Entry #3

Hi Michael,

You'll be pleased to know that I've stopped eating those humungous chocolate chip cookies that I'd often have for an afternoon energy boost. I'm also now using milk in my tea instead of half-and-half. What sacrifice! What do you think about substituting a rice cake for my afternoon cookie? In general, I think I'm eating too many sugary, high-carbohydrate foods. And not enough protein.

Well, I managed to walk a few times over the past four days, but I've had no other form of exercise. I actually carried my youngest son (on my shoulders) for a thirty-minute walk at the Broadmore Audubon Reserve. Doing this speaks to the heart of why I would like to be more fit—to be able to spend more time with my sons and keep up with them when I do!

More regarding the before and after pictures . . . I hope that my willingness to bare my fifty-year-old, sadly neglected body will inspire readers to face their situation honestly and see that, like me, they are not a lost cause. People tell me that I look good in a jacket and tie, but the fact is that clothes can hide a multitude of sins. If you want to know what kind of shape you're *really* in, stand in front of a full-length mirror naked and take a good, hard look. And I can't deny reality when it comes to picking up my kids, playing with them, or hiking the John Muir Trail, so I might as well accept the truth and use it as a platform for change.

Did I tell you that I have some weights and a Universal machine in my basement? In addition to this, we have a recumbent bike and a treadmill. My wife uses both regularly, but I never go near them (Michael, your work is cut out for you!). I'm thinking that I'll use what we have here at the house and forgo a gym membership (for convenience). Any thoughts?

> 66
>
> If you want to know what kind of shape you're *really* in, stand in front of a full-length mirror naked and take a good, hard look.
>
> 99

Journal Entry #4

Hi Michael,

Okay, regarding an exercise program, here's what I've come up with. I'll join Gold's Gym and train there twice a week. During the week (at lunchtime), I'll go to the gym at the hotel near where I work. Finally, I'll augment this by training at home three times a week. One day I'll use heavy weights for my upper body and light weights for my lower (the next day, I'll do the opposite). Then, to increase my endurance, I'll do three sets with a light weight, performing twenty-five reps or more. Then I'll do two sets at 90 percent of my max (around seven or eight reps) to increase my strength.

With this hybrid arrangement, I can train at two convenient locations. For an aerobic workout, I'll walk, ride a bike, or use the treadmill in my basement. I'll stretch at night as a complement to the weight training.

Let me try this out before we meet. If it's working, great. If not, I'll ask for help. Sound good?

Reply from Michael

Hey! Who's the trainer here, anyway? And what is my role in this process? Casual observer?

Chet, this is way too much! Left to your own devices, you'd be flat on your back for a week!

I'll tell you all about reps, sets, etc., when I see you, but for the time being, please be patient. I can see that one of your UFOs (unidentified fitness obstacles) is misconceptions about exercise, based on your past experience with training. Let's talk about this.

I know that you want to start early so you'll look good in your Speedo for the photo shoot, but let's not jump the gun here. You'll be well on your way very soon!

CHET

Weight, girth measurements, and body fat percentage, before:

Height: 6'2½"
Weight: 212 lbs.
Chest: 42½"
Waist: 40¼"
Hips: 43"
Upper thighs: 24" (L), 23½" (R)
Calves: 15½" (L), 15¾" (R)
Ankles: 9¼" (L), 9½" (R)
Upper arms: 13¾" (L), 14" (R)
Forearms: 11½" (L), 12" (R)
Wrists: 7" (L), 7" (R)
Body fat: 29.5%

Journal Entry #5

Hi Michael,
You're right. It is too much. Good grief, maybe that's my problem?
I keep thinking that I'm still twenty years old. Or training for the
Olympics! Okay, I'll keep eating bonbons until I meet you on the 20th.

I guess I need to read your book. It's by my nightstand
(honestly!). All right, I'm going to read it now. Talk to you soon!

Journal Entry #6

Hi Michael,
I decided today that building igloos is pretty good aerobic exercise.
Talk about exertion! My kids loved it.

I'm going away on a trip tomorrow, but I'm bringing my walking
shoes. Looking forward to our official start. See you soon!

Journal Entry #7

Hi Michael,
Good thing we didn't start this week. I've put on 5 pounds! Help! I'm
going backward!

Week 1—Journal Entry #8

Hi Michael!
I really enjoyed our time together. Thanks for all your advice. I'm off
to a good start with my diet. I'm totally psyched (and starved!).

Impressions of the Photo Shoot and Consultation

I really liked Jack (your photographer). He really put me at ease
(although I was not particularly nervous to begin with). Besides
being grateful that the photographs would be taken by a professional, I was glad there wasn't an emphasis on unflattering "before"
pictures. We did only what was needed to show my starting point—
nothing more. It was honest and straightforward.

Regarding the photo shoot, one of the things I enjoyed most was
unexpected. It was really great to chat with a couple of interesting

guys who live and work with passion. I don't often have the opportunity to compare notes with other guys unless it has something to do with business. That's a pity—that I don't make time for male friendships. I intend for that to change. I've just been too busy with work, not to mention exhausted!

I also enjoyed getting to know you and fielding your questions. And hearing your responses to my questions. It was a learning experience, and I enjoy that kind of thing. I look forward to more of the same!

Week 1—Journal Entry #9

Hi Michael!

Put a checkmark by day one! Here's what I did today:

I worked out on the treadmill at 9:00 P.M. (three-minute warm-up, followed by twenty minutes maintaining my target heart rate). I also did some extra "belly crunches" (I'd like to get a bit ahead of the game in that department!).

You asked me to tell you if I had any food cravings. Peanut butter. I always make the kids peanut butter and jelly sandwiches. I really wanted one today!

Regarding the diet, a major plus is that Ande (my wife) knows a lot about food prep and is a wonderful chef. Yesterday we bought a food scale and stocked our shelves with healthy food. Here's what I had today:

Breakfast
    1 tangerine
    1 serving turkey
    1 cup coffee w/1 tablespoon 2% milk

Lunch
    1 serving tofu (pan fried without oil, seasoned)
    1 serving tuna (water packed)
    1 serving sunflower seeds (raw)
    1 serving almonds (4 nuts, raw)
    1 cup green tea

Before-Dinner Snack
  1 piece of rye toast

Dinner
  1 salad (romaine w/nonfat dressing and seven miniature tomatoes)
  1 serving scallops
  1 serving swordfish
  1 serving winter squash

I can't say this isn't a stretch for me. I normally eat a lot more and almost never hold back on dessert. But it wasn't that difficult, either. For most of the day I was aware of being on a diet, but not all that stressed about it.

  Well, that's it for day one. Hope you had a great weekend.

Week 1—Journal Entry #10

Hi Michael!
I had more trouble today (mentally) with the diet. It seems that my grazing habits involve more than just satisfying my hunger. They provide a break from my routine. I miss this. So, I'm going to continue to take breaks, but instead of eating, I'll drop in on some of my favorite people for a few minutes each day, or have tea instead of a cookie.

  Today I worked out for twenty minutes again (on the treadmill). Tomorrow I start with the weights. I'm looking forward to it!

  I had more energy today. I didn't experience the "crash" that I normally have around 3:00 in the afternoon. That was nice—and unexpected.

Week 2—Journal Entry #11

Hi Michael,
Thanks for the redirection! I started my weight training routine today and realized that I need to allow more time (right now the routine is about forty-five minutes long). Second, I had difficulty maintaining good form. I'll report in greater detail on my next go-round with the weights.

I weighed in tonight at about 209, down slightly from 210. That's about it. I hope things are going well with the other folks. Talk to you soon.

Week 2—Journal Entry #12

Hi Michael!

I hear you regarding the futility of weighing myself every day. Thanks!

This morning I spent twenty-five minutes on the treadmill. I got a nice sweat going. I can't believe how much my energy level has increased during the day! Already! Now I walk briskly wherever I go and I no longer feel so fatigued. I feel great!

Believe it or not, Andrea has lost 4 pounds since I started the program. She is eating the same way I do now, and it's really paying off. As you might imagine, she is very happy about this! By the way, she wants me to add that she has been making great meals and been a very supportive wife!

> 66
>
> I can't believe how much my energy level has increased during the day! Already! Now I walk briskly wherever I go and I no longer feel so fatigued. I feel great!
>
> 99

Week 3—Journal Entry #13

Hi Michael!

I've been holding my own with the diet. All has been well—except for one minor setback.

Saturday morning I pulled a muscle in my upper back. Did I do it lifting weights? Not on your life. I was playing with Mattie (my four-year-old son) on the couch. I can still move okay, and I'm not in terrible pain, but it looks like I won't be lifting anything, at least for a few more days.

Here's the good news . . . I've already lost 4 pounds! Today I was able to tighten my belt one extra notch (an exciting unit of measurement), and it felt great. I have a long way to go, but one thing is certain . . . this diet *works*, and I love what I'm seeing! Now I just have to get on track with my weight training.

Hope all is well with you and Cheryl.

> 66
>
> Today I was able to tighten my belt one extra notch (an exciting unit of measurement), and it felt great. I have a long way to go, but one thing is certain . . . this diet works, and I love what I'm seeing!
>
> 99

Note to Reader

Insulin instability was one of Chet's top UFOs. Because of this, he started with Plan B (see page 193).

Hi Michael,
Weekend update . . . I noticed during my last workout that
my legs felt much stronger! And I'm now down to 205 pounds!
Looking (and feeling) good!

Week 5—Journal Entry #15

Hi Michael,
Uh-ohhh. I hear ya. Guilty as charged. I promise that from now on I'll
be in touch more often. Meanwhile, here's an update:

One of the most recent and best changes I've experienced is
a feeling of "lightness" (both mentally and physically). I'll give you an
example of what I mean. We have a three-level house. It used to be
that when I went from the first to the third floor, I felt like I was
wearing lead shoes. It took tremendous effort just to pick up my
feet. Now I walk up the stairs with no problem at all! It no longer
occurs to me that I'm doing anything difficult. What a great feeling!

Here's another example. Last weekend we met some friends who
have two boys the same age as ours. We took all the kids to the
pond to go sleigh riding. I must have walked up and down the hill at
least fifteen or twenty times, often with Mattie, my youngest, in
tow. I had absolutely no problem at all! Being there for the kids . . .
that's the best payoff of all!

I weigh 204 pounds today (down from 212 when I started). This is
in spite of the fact that toward the end of last week I went off the
diet a bit. Anyway, I'm still pleased that I've lost 8 pounds. I've
gained some muscle, too (I can tell).

A peculiarity in my "transformation" is that I seem to be losing
fat from the top down. For example, I still have a gut, although it's
smaller than when I began. In contrast, my chest and arms are looking trim and my strength is improving rapidly.

As far as my diet goes, everything is good. I no longer experience
cravings and seem to feel full eating much less food. One of the keys
to my success is Andrea—she does a wonderful job creating meals
that are in keeping with my plan. She's following the diet, too, and
get this . . . she has lost 9 pounds! She looks terrific! Today she said
"I wish I had known about this a long time ago."

> **"**
> I must have walked
> up and down the hill
> at least fifteen or
> twenty times, often
> with Mattie, my
> youngest, in tow.
> I had absolutely no
> problem at all! Being
> there for the kids . . .
> that's the best
> payoff of all!
> **"**

CHET'S UFOs

Work Addiction
Poor Life/Time Management
Insulin Instability
Low Testosterone
DHEA Imbalance
Amino Acid Deficiency
Cortisol Imbalance
Adrenal Burnout
Perfectionism
Improper Food Combining

Week 6—Journal Entry #16

Hi Michael!
My top two UFOs make complete sense. My work addiction is hard to deny. And just this morning Andrea said, "You have trouble managing time." So that one makes sense, too. I love to take on projects, but I get so focused on what I'm doing that everything else in my life gets ignored. I crave the intellectual challenge of solving a problem. I don't know what this says about me, but I do know that it isn't conducive to maintaining a normal schedule.

Week 7—Journal Entry #17

Hi Michael!
Let me start off by saying that I am now 200 pounds! I am amazed! I even went off my diet (two days ago at Hunter's Cub Scout Award Dinner). Dinner was pasta with meatballs. I was a madman (my Polish genes kicked in at the sight of meatballs) and I decided to go for it. Aside from that incident, I've been pretty good about sticking to the plan.

I have not done any weight training since we met at the health club last weekend. But if I work out today, I'll be back on track.

It's been a killer ten days at the office, but things should lighten up soon. Once they do, I hope to be more consistent with my workouts. Until then, I'll do the best I can. As someone once said:

"A crooked row plowed is better than a straight row unplowed!"
Talk with you soon!

Week 8—Journal Entry #18

Hi Michael,

Well, it's been a full week since I've checked in. I've not been doing as well. I've been thinking a lot about why this is the case. I really, truly want to stick with the program (like during the first few weeks), but for some reason I haven't been able to. My thoughts are as follows:

1. I'm a perfectionist. When I can't do something "right," I "priori-tize" by neglecting what I don't have the time or resources to do perfectly.
2. I'm not a good "macro" planner. I think I know what I need to do (intellectually), but I don't. I'm not entirely sure why. I think I have more of an artist mentality.
3. I've made my job my first priority. In my mind (and heart) it's my family and health, but in practice, it's not the case.
4. I have a lot of guilt about my failure to perform. I feel like I'm letting myself down (and letting you down, too). The result? I repress. I become less creative and less effective. Time slips by, like water through sand, and I don't get a lot of things done.

> 66
>
> I've made my job my first priority. In my mind (and heart) it's my family and health, but in practice, it's not the case.
>
> 99

By the way, I am now 199 pounds! I haven't been less than 200 since before I turned forty years old. So even though I haven't followed the program to the letter, I'm amazed at what I've achieved.

Note to Reader

It was right around this time that Chet discovered he'd lost his job. This, as you might imagine, wasn't conducive to staying on track. The loss of a very good income (with a wife and two kids to support) put Chet under lots of pressure to find a new job right away. For the next five weeks, he faced some facts about how he was living his life. Spending more time with his family made him aware of what matters most—taking care of himself and spending more time with his wife and kids.

This kind of hardship often makes people start to ignore their health. Or overeat "comfort foods" in order to deal with all the stress. But the best way to deal with stress, I've found, is focusing *more* on your health. It took Chet a while to realize this, but he made great strides once he did.

Week 12—Journal Entry #19

Hi Michael:

Some thoughts:

At the start of this program, my main goal was to feel better and get fit. I have to say . . . unequivocally . . . that I've realized that goal. Case in point:

Yesterday I walked five laps around our pond. I felt great. In fact, I felt so good that I jogged the last lap and a half. And as I was jogging I made a discovery . . . I "feel good" when I run! I haven't had that feeling for well over fifteen years!

Second example. Today Andrea and I took the kids to the Patriot's Parade in Lexington. Her dad was marching in the Marine Corps band. Anyhow, after a while, we were able to see him as he marched by. The kids really loved seeing "Poppa" playing the trombone in the parade. So we ran to where the parade would end so we could see him again. Again, I felt just great. Running along with the kids felt like it took no effort at all!

CHET

Weight, girth measurements, and body fat percentage, after 12 weeks:

Height: 6'2½"
Weight: 191 lbs. (−21 lbs.)
Chest: 41" (−1½")
Waist: 36¾" (−3½")
Hips: 40" (−3")
Upper thighs: 23¼" (L), 23" (R) (−¾", −½")
Calves: 15¼" (L), 15¼" (R) (−¼", −½")
Ankles: 9" (L), 9¼" (R) (−¼", −¼")
Upper arms: 13¼" (L), 13½" (R) (−½", −½")
Forearms: 11¼" (L), 11¾" (R) (−¼", −¼")
Wrists: 7" (L), 7" (R) (no change)
Total inches lost: 12"
Body fat: 20% (−9.5%)

Have I reached every one of my goals? The honest answer is no. But I was naive when I started and had no sense of pace. I'm much more in tune with my body now, and clear about what it can do. I've lacked this kind of awareness for at least the past thirty years.

When I started the program, we joked about me getting a six-pack. Believe it or not, I feel like I'm almost there! The only downside is that I'll have to go out and buy new pants again. And have my jackets tailored. But it's well worth the cost!

Regarding my lab results . . . for the most part, everything was within normal range. My total cholesterol was 170 (when I started it was 230!). My blood pressure was good too (120/70). So there have been measurable results. The only area of concern was (you guessed it) my testosterone level. It was 260—the lower range of normal (the normal range is 241 to 827 ng/dl). Not enough to justify an intervention now, but something to keep an eye on (and perhaps, test once again).

I still have some negative feelings about exercise, but this program has helped me confront them. In college, I threw the javelin and had Olympic hopes. But I gave up my chance to compete to focus on doing better in school. When I abandoned my dream of competing in the Olympics, I put the idea of training (for anything) totally out of my mind. And I always compared myself (later) to who, and what, I once had been.

To the reader, I would say two things: (1) I wouldn't have done nearly as well if it wasn't for this program (this is not a gratuitous plug, it's just a statement of fact); and (2) it was harder than I thought it would be, especially mentally. You *really will* confront UFOs that you don't even know you have. After all, if you're out of shape (and have been for a while) it's going to take more than a whim of will for you to turn this around. Now I can't imagine getting in shape any other way.

> 66
>
> When I started the program, we joked about me getting a six-pack. Believe it or not, I feel like I'm almost there!
>
> 99

CHAPTER TEN

L'TANYA

I have to remind myself: I will not do this program, or
anything else, perfectly. And I won't give up when I don't.

L'Tanya
    Age: 42
    Height: 5'5"
    Weight: 250 lbs.
    Occupation: Life Coach, Writer

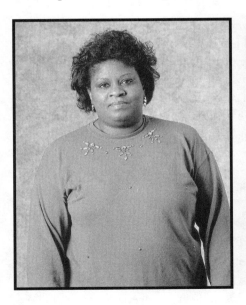 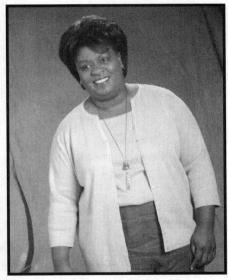

Excerpt from letter:

Five years ago, my twenty-month-old son and I survived being struck by a
tractor-trailer truck, traveling 56 miles per hour. Eight people were killed,
including my husband. I have successfully worked through much of my
anxiety, depression, survivor's guilt, and post-traumatic stress. However, my

body does not reflect the work I've done internally. To me, this is a sign that there is more work to be done.

Journal Entry #1

I can hardly believe that I've been chosen to participate in this project! When I received the news, I clapped my hands and said, "Yes!" Lenny (my six-year-old son) asked, "What is it, Mommy?" I said, "Mommy is going to be in a book!" Then he said, "Mommy, you can't fit in a book!" Kids! I laughed all the way home.

Journal Entry #2

> 66
>
> I have always been lonely. Always. And over and over again, as people come into my life and leave I feel like a piece of me goes with them. Is my overeating an attempt to fill the void?
>
> 99

I've been thinking a lot about my life lately. I've been thinking about all of my destructive behavior—eating, drinking . . . whatever. What feelings have I been trying to avoid? I think I know. I've probably always known. I'm lonely.

I have always been lonely. Always. And over and over again, as people come into my life and leave I feel like a piece of me goes with them. Is my overeating an attempt to fill the void?

It's so much easier for me to do things for others (as opposed to for myself). For example, I would do anything for my son and my mother. And how many men have I said that to? "I would do anything for you." God!

I want to start taking better care of myself. I don't want to die having never really lived. Like they said in that movie *Bounce*, it's not brave if you're not scared. For once in my life, I'm going to be brave.

Journal Entry #3

> 66
>
> The scale at the doctor's office always reads something different—higher—than my scale. I actually asked if I could stand on it facing *backward*.
>
> 99

Today I went to the doctor to get a physical. I had shared with a friend how long it had been since I had a pap smear. But I didn't tell her why it had been so long: my fear of being weighed!

My doctor has never lectured me about my weight, but I was still anxious about seeing her. Thank God she was booked until January. I had to make an appointment with her assistant. "Good," I thought, "she doesn't know me."

The scale at the doctor's office always reads something different—higher—than my scale. I actually asked if I could stand on it facing *backward*. I almost glanced at what she wrote down, but I knew it would make me depressed.

Getting a physical was a major accomplishment for me. I could have put it off indefinitely. How many times have I said to myself that I would get my act together once I lost weight? I say it all the time. It's like I can't start living until I do.

Reply from Michael

Hi L'Tanya,
Regarding the story you told (in your introductory letter) about losing your husband in an auto accident . . . is this when you began to gain weight? This is a common occurrence when people experience this kind of loss. Many people use food to fill the void (so to speak) and gain weight to avoid relationships (that may result in another loss). Does any of this strike a chord?

Journal Entry #4

Michael,
To answer your question, I was 10 pounds away from my goal weight when I met my husband. I got married for the wrong reason. I was lonely (surprise). I knew it was wrong from the start. So, I started gaining weight immediately because I was unhappy.

After the accident, I probably did gain weight, but I don't remember anything significant. But I do believe that I've been trying to prevent painful experiences. And that I've been using food (for comfort) and gaining fat (to hide). I know that I have an abandonment issue, so it's true that I often don't want anyone to get too close to me, even though I'm *painfully* lonely.

This is going to be an interesting time for me in many respects. I recently started seeing someone—someone who actually seems to care more about who I am than what I look like. But I don't trust it.

Journal Entry #5

I had a chance to see *Oprah* on Tuesday. Dr. Phil was talking about something called "the get real challenge." He asked the question, "What do you want for your life?" Then he explained how to find the answer. He said when you get it, you'll know it in your gut.

So what do I want? I want to be in a relationship where I feel loved. I want to *feel* loved. I want to love *myself*.

Journal Entry #6

Yesterday, I felt completely empty . . . passionless and alone. This is why I overeat and *overeverything*—to fill this empty vessel. This is how I feel and it hurts.

I'm so tired of feeling this way. I want to stop hiding myself. I want to live an "authentic" life.

Journal Entry #7

There's a battle waging inside me—like my mind is at war with my gut. My gut has this "default setting" (like a computer) and I don't know how to reset it. My mind says, "You've got so much to offer." My default says no one is ever going to love me. Mind: Every time somebody leaves, God is clearing space for something, or someone, better. Default: They all leave. Mind: Good friends are priceless. Default: The only relationship that matters is a romantic one. Mind: I am intelligent and have the potential to accomplish great things. Default: If there's no one to share my achievements with, what does it matter? Mind: I am a patient and caring mother. Default: I have failed to provide a home for my son with two caring parents.

Wow. No wonder I'm feeling stuck! Will all of this ever stop?

Week 1—Journal Entry #8

Well, I started the program. It is definitely something I have to ease into. The past two days have been okay, but not great.

Last night, I was reading *The Dark Side of the Light Chasers* by Debbie Ford. The more I read, the angrier I got—even though it was enlightening. I've been "closing doors" for years! No wonder I've never reached my potential! I realize that I've never forgiven myself for *any-thing* (nor have I forgiven anyone else!). I live in the past a lot and it pisses me off because I've missed a lifetime of present moments. I have a word-for-word memory of events in the past that have really hurt me. They are hardwired into my brain.

When I was eleven or twelve, somebody told me that I had a really big toe. That was the first time I remember thinking I was different. I closed a door. In tenth grade, someone said my legs were shaped like ice cream cones. Message—don't show my legs—close another door. In high school, I was the cocaptain of my cheerleading team. Whenever I could, I would wear pants underneath my cheerleading outfit. My boyfriend and his friends used to call me the "black bull" because I was dark skinned and had thick legs. Close another door. That guy (my boyfriend) had a real issue with people who were overweight (I wasn't). He always seemed to be dissatisfied with the way I looked. Something had to be wrong with me. Close another door. When I lived in New York, a guy I was dating asked if I used to be a man. What? I look like a *man*? Close that door fast! I was once a really good tap and jazz dancer but was always self-conscious. I remember taking a class with a lot of professional dancers. After one of the classes, a guy walks up to me and grabs my shoulders with both hands. He didn't say why he did that, but to me it meant "You've got big shoulders, hide them." And of course there was the time that one of my coworkers had a baby. I remember going to her house. She hadn't returned home yet, but her husband was there. He was saying that she needed to lose weight. I said, "I think she

---

L'TANYA

Weight, girth measurements, and body fat percentage, before:

Height: 5'5"
Weight: 250 lbs.
Chest (bust): 50¼"
Waist: 43"
Hips: 50½"
Upper thighs: 30¾" (L), 31½" (R)
Calves: 17¾" (L), 18" (R)
Ankles: 9¼" (L), 9½" (R)
Upper arms: 16" (L), 16" (R)
Forearms: 13" (L), 13¼" (R)
Wrists: 7¼" (L), 7¼" (R)
Body fat: 43%

---

looks fine." I will never forget what he said. He said, "Yeah, well look at you." I didn't say a word.

So, at forty-two, I won't wear shorts. I won't wear anything sleeveless. Never mind that I have the muscle tone of my father—the kind of body that responds beautifully and quickly to exercise. Never mind that I was a captain of two cheerleading squads in high school. Never mind that with a little more training, I had the potential to be a professional Broadway dancer. But I missed my chance. And I don't get a do-over. Not in this lifetime at least.

I am so angry. I am angry at all the hurt, but mainly I'm angry that I allowed people to hurt me. Maybe this is my "shadow" (or one of my shadows) that has never surfaced before? All this time, I was thinking I was a stress eater or that I ate because I was lonely. Now I'm starting to see how much my anger affects what I do. Since I'm the one whom I'm most angry at, I wonder if I'm trying to punish myself? I don't really know right now . . .

Week 1—Journal Entry #9

I have all these things running through my head. I read the first chapter of Michael's book (*When Working Out Isn't Working Out*). He mentioned an incident that occurred when he was very young that changed his life. It made me think about one of my classes. A student was talking about the idea of "doing" as opposed to "trying." I wonder how much of my life I've spent trying to do something. I try to lose weight. I try to eat right. I try to meet interesting people. I try to organize my house. I'm always trying but never doing. Michael didn't try to get fit—he decided he would and he did. So, I'm going to stop "trying."

I realize that I need to get organized. I did a much better job grocery shopping yesterday than I did last week. This week, I'm going to eat (and exercise) according to my plan—not some half-hearted version of it. I'm not going to try, I'm just going to do it!

Week 2—Journal Entry #10

Michael,
Plans have changed quickly. My mother has been hospitalized and is

Week 2—Journal Entry #11

Michael,
Thanks for your call. My mother did come through her surgery well,
though she will be in ICU for a while. She's got age (sixty-five years
old) and a strong heart on her side, but diabetes, neuropathy,
hypertension, obesity, and a kidney disorder will not make her
recovery any easier. Here's the gift—now I *really* want to be healthy!

Week 3—Journal Entry #12

Michael,
My mother is still in the hospital but out of ICU. This has knocked
me for a loop. I am a single mother and an only child, so I have no one
to lean on. My son has been out of school for winter break, so I have
not been able to concentrate on anything. I am exhausted, stressed,
and overwhelmed.

But hey, life happens! So, I will journal about what it has been like
for me during the past few weeks. Seeing my mother like this is
heartbreaking and I want to avoid the same fate. In a way, it has
made me even more determined to succeed.

Week 3—Journal Entry #13

After triple bypass surgery and a two-and-a-half-week stay in the
hospital, Ma is coming home. For the past three weeks, I feel like
I've been in a coma. This experience has reminded me that I am a
single parent with an only child and I'm living my life *alone*. Until this
moment, I don't think I realized how worn out and stressed out I
was. But a funny thing happened on the way to a nervous breakdown.
My mindset completely changed! When I first started the project,
I felt like I was being stripped of everything that was familiar. In my
mind I was saying, "Well, they're not going to take everything away.
I'm going to keep my coffee or my whatever." I realize now that I
was fighting with *myself*.

> 66
> When I first started
> the project, I felt like
> I was being stripped
> of everything that
> was familiar. In my
> mind I was saying,
> "Well, they're not
> going to take every-
> thing away. I'm going
> to keep my coffee or
> my whatever." I realize
> now that I was fight-
> ing with *myself*.
> 99

Something has shifted for me. I'm sure it was seeing my mother so vulnerable and sick. I don't want to end up the same way. So yesterday I was even more mindful of what I was putting into my mouth. Instead of focusing on what's being "taken" from me, I'm just going to keep things simple. All I have to do is follow the plan. Don't think about it, don't analyze it, don't criticize it. Just do it. It's actually less stressful that way.

I didn't exercise yesterday. I've got to get to the gym. I will.

Week 3—Journal Entry #14

Eating healthy is getting easier. I had a *moment* today. While grocery shopping, I must have passed the donuts and Trix cereal boxes at least five times. It didn't phase me one bit. But later, in my kitchen, hiding on the top shelf, way, way back in the deep, dark recesses of a crowded cabinet, I detected some semi-sweet chocolate pieces. I thought, "O-o-oh, chocolate pieces!" I didn't touch them. But I craved them. Why?

At about 7:00 P.M. I dozed and I had one of my flashbacks. Gosh, this is the second time I've had this particular one! I'm driving and all of a sudden a car crosses right in front of me. I'm not sure if I hit it or not. Because of my history, the idea of getting into a car crash really scares me. So when I woke up, I *really* wanted something sweet. I went to the cabinet, weighed out one-third of a cup of chocolate pieces and devoured them. Then I started thinking about what was going through my mind before I did this. I realized that I eat when I'm tired and anxious. I had never (really) put this together before.

I haven't been able to exercise this week—yet. I have been so, so tired. I think that with everything that is going on right now, I've been on autopilot. It has been hard for me to do anything, let alone go to the gym. I've also been napping a lot. I never take naps, but I must need them. But at least I'm sticking to my diet. For the most part . . .

Week 4—Journal Entry #15

I am getting some real gifts of insight during my mother's illness and recovery. People are there to help if you ask and *tell them what you need!* I was talking to a friend the other day and I was explaining what my schedule was like. I told her that I was in over my head and I felt like I was slowly drowning. I think that was the first time I admitted that to myself—or to anyone!

Week 4—Journal Entry #16

I finally completed Michael's UFO test. *Wow!* I had an inkling that something was going on, but I was never able to put it all together the way this test did. I'm almost finished with the assessment, but I can't wait to get Michael's feedback.

Cheryl's classes have been great. I'm going to the gym today when the physical therapist comes to Ma's house, which is the agreement I made with Cheryl.

As I'm writing this, I'm listening to music. This is the first time I've written in my journal and listened to music at the same time. I forgot how much I love music and how relaxing it is to me. I've forgotten about a lot of things I enjoy.

I've been trying to figure out what the deal is with writing in a food diary, keeping an exercise log, exercising, and sticking to my diet. It feels like so many pieces have to come together all at once. Keeping a food journal is no big deal when I'm eating right. But it's a pain when I'm not. Hmmm . . . I just figured out why. Duh!

I've also been comparing myself (a lot) to the other participants in the project. I keep thinking that everyone else is doing a lot better than me. This is one of the reasons why the teleclasses have been so helpful. It helps to hear that I'm not the only one who is struggling. I was beating myself up and thinking that I didn't deserve to be involved in the project. But I'm realizing that this is a starting point, not an end point. I am learning so much about myself. And what I've learned, and will learn, will benefit me for the rest of my life.

> 66
>
> Keeping a food journal is no big deal when I'm eating right. But it's a pain when I'm not. Hmmm . . . I just figured out why. Duh!
>
> 99

Week 4—Journal Entry #17

Whoa! Discovering my UFOs is kind of like a "good" slap in the face! Seeing them spelled out like this is extremely helpful. I know my body image sucks. Winter always sucks. I've always suspected that I've suffered from depression, and of course, low self-esteem. But I never really thought about ADD. My son has many of the same issues.

L'TANYA'S UFOs

Seasonal Affective Disorder (SAD)

Perfectionism

"Askaphobia" (Fear of Asking for Help)

Attention Deficit Disorder (ADD)

Cortisol Imbalance

Sleep Apnea

Body Dysmorphic Disorder (BDD)

Sleep Debt

Dysthymia (Low-Grade Depression)

Diet Misconceptions

Maybe he is modeling me?

Michael suggested that I speak to my doctor about taking Wellbutrin, a medication that addresses ADD as well as depression. I'm not opposed to this. In fact, I've taken Prozac off and on for the past ten years. I was actually taking it a year ago but decided to stop. I didn't want to be on an antidepressant for the rest of my life.

Okay, so now that I have this information, what do I do with it? I'm nervous just thinking about it!

On another note, it seems like I always find my motivation from a source outside myself. Just two years ago, I lost weight just because I wanted to get someone's attention. If there was a contest to win, a man to impress, or an event to go to, I'd be inspired to try harder. I guess what this means is that improving my health is not a good enough reason. How sad . . .

Week 5—Journal Entry #18 (to Cheryl Richardson)

Hi Cheryl,

I wanted to let you know that I spoke with Lenny's great uncle Stevie. He said that he would be glad to pick him up every Monday from school and spend some time with him! Lenny will also have a chance to spend Monday evenings with his paternal grandmother (Uncle Stevie's sister). She's been really wanting to work with him on his reading.

I've talked to Michael about some of the challenges I'm facing. I'm wondering if you could also advise. I think I "need" a deadline/

contest/whatever to have as a goal. Michael suggested that I hang a sign in my office that says, "*I am the most important reason to improve my health*" (in other words, *not* some superficial goal). I've also made signs that say, "I do complete work" and "I do consistent work."

When I think about keeping an exercise log and food diary, writing in my journal, eating well (all the time), and exercising, it feels like so much to do. When I dig deeper, I think that having to do all these things feels like a loss of freedom. That's as far as I get with the digging.

Week 5—Journal Entry #19

Michael,
I worked out on Friday and it felt *good*. I would like to make weekly commitments to you. It seems to work for me. So, I hearby commit to going to the gym three times this week.

Reply from Michael

Hi L'Tanya,
This is your conscience speaking . . . have you called your doctor yet? Let's not put this off any longer, okay? Pretty soon, it'll be twelve weeks and it would be a shame if we didn't address some of your physical issues/UFOs before the project concludes.
I'm thrilled that you're stepping up your efforts and that from now on you'll be making regular weekly commitments. Good for you!
Also, please let me know when you receive your light box. I'll need to tell you how to use it.

Week 5—Journal Entry #20

Michael,
Just wanted to let you know that I received the light box today, although I haven't opened the box. I'll give my doctor a call and schedule an appointment re: Wellbutrin.

Reply from Michael

Hi L'Tanya,
Here is your bright-light prescription: (a) set up the light so that it's

about 2 to 3 feet from your eyes (directly in front of you for now); (b) at first, don't use the light for any longer than thirty minutes (it might give you headaches if you do); (c) don't stare at the light—instead, glance at it (briefly) every twenty to thirty seconds; and (d) report in about how you feel within the next few days.

Week 6—Journal Entry #21

> **"**
> Surprisingly, discovering that I might have ADD was *encouraging.* I'm usually the first one to say that ADD is overdiagnosed, but based on my history and behavior, it all makes perfect sense!
> **"**

Happy birthday to me! I feel like I've been given a huge gift. Michael sent me the results of my UFO test, which revealed some very interesting things. My highest scores were SAD, ADD, perfectionism, and body image issues. The "gift" was that it finally gave me something to "grab on to." Up until this point, all I knew was that I didn't feel good and was always tired. I kept beating myself up, thinking that I was lazy and undisciplined. Surprisingly, discovering that I might have ADD was *encouraging.* I'm usually the first one to say that ADD is overdiagnosed, but based on my history and behavior, it all makes perfect sense! Once I received the test results, I started thinking more about how I operate. I consider myself a "brilliant scatterbrain" (to myself). Typically, I read five books at once (and it takes me a year to finish just one). Also, I can never seem to get my house in order. I'll start in one area, but then I get distracted, or bored, and go to another before I finish the one I started with. So as a result, nothing gets completed.

I think what excites me most about seeing my results laid out in a top ten list is that now I *really* know what to address. And I can stop beating myself up. It's exciting to think that once these issues are addressed, there will be a light at the end of the tunnel.

Today, I started my light therapy. I like it a lot. I also like it because I can do other things at the same time. This morning, I was taking a class on the phone while I sat in front of my light box. The next step is to see a doctor.

Week 6—Journal Entry #22

Bright-light therapy is good for me! It is the one thing so far that I have been doing consistently (well, except for yesterday).

Michael sent out an update on all of the project participants.

I feel terrible. I always compare myself to others and feel like I come out on the bottom. I guess it's the perfectionist thing rearing its ugly head *again*. What if I don't lose as much as the other people? What if their pictures look great and mine look horrible? I can "what if" until the cows come home. If I let myself.

I like Cheryl's idea of doing one new thing to improve my health/fitness every day. She said that it could be as simple as carrying a water bottle. This makes a lot of sense to me and shouldn't be hard to do.

The good news is that I feel like I'm on the verge of some really big improvements. I guess everyone works differently. Up until now, I would *want* to follow the program, but there was a gap between wanting to and actually doing it. This has been very frustrating. I've felt like something was wrong with me.

At least now I have *time* to exercise. This week, in particular, I have nothing on my schedule that could interfere. I had a talk with my mother about not wanting to be on call anymore—about going to run her errands on *my* schedule. She was fine with it. I took a stand and cleared my schedule. Now what am I going to do?

Week 7—Journal Entry #23

I have trouble scheduling time for myself. So, Ray (the sweetest man I've ever met) helped me plan a schedule for the week. For once, I actually made room for *me*. Me first!!! Once I did that, I had a great day. Everything seemed to line up.

Then there's the perfectionist thing. I'm all or nothing; black or white. I struggle to find the middle ground in almost every area of my life. So, I have to remind myself: I will not do this program, or anything else, perfectly. And I won't give up when I don't.

I feel like for once in my life, I'm starting to give myself a break. I've been feeling tired, probably because I've been depressed. But it could also be my hectic schedule and, of course, not sleeping well. Heck, beating myself up all the time is tiring, too!

The UFO test results and light therapy have been critical for me. They've given me tools and wings!

I hope that I can keep building on this feeling. Michael says let today be a template . . .

Week 7—Journal Entry #24

Michael,

I already went to the gym today!!! Can you believe it? Two days in a row! I did a ten-minute warm-up, some lower-body work, and fifteen minutes on the bike. I'll E-mail my food diary later.

Thanks for everything!

Week 7—Journal Entry #25

> 66
>
> I have to remind myself: I will not do this program, or anything else, perfectly. And I won't give up when I don't.
>
> 99

Valentine's Day! Ray and I agreed not to get each other candy since we're both changing our eating habits. So, we didn't. It was so nice to go out and have someone actually buy me something for Valentine's Day. I can't remember the last time that happened. It ended up not being a classic romantic date. We went to a restaurant where there was a three-hour wait. No food tastes that good! So we went to a pizza parlor. Okay, I ate pizza, but the good news is that I didn't beat myself up. I just said, I'll get back on track tomorrow. Ms. Black or White finally found gray!

I saw my doctor today. Before I stepped on the scale, I had a moment of "Oh no, should I stand on it backward?" I don't do scales! But today, for the first time in a long time, I actually got on it facing forward. I even looked! When the doctor saw me, we talked about the project, SAD, ADD, and the fact that I've had three colds in the past four months and have been feeling pretty yucky—consistently. Well, it's not a cold after all. It's a sinus infection. She said colds generally last for about a week and the symptoms disappear, but sinus infections last longer. Another blessing . . . another answer (she prescribed antibiotics). We talked about SAD and the cyclical nature of depression. I was a little ambivalent about taking medication because I'm doing so well with the light therapy and I feel pretty good now (emotionally). With regard to the ADD issue, she wanted to know if I felt scattered as a child. I don't know when it started, but I know that for a long time now, it has been a real problem for me. I left with a prescription for Wellbutrin. But here's the best thing . . . (drumroll, please) . . . I lost weight! How about that! I actually faced the "scale God" and received some encouraging news!

I started taking my antibiotic this evening and already I feel better. I didn't feel too good writing that check at the pharmacy, though. This is another part about being self-employed, overweight, and depressed that I hate. It's hard to get health insurance. On Wednesday, I talked to a new insurance company about getting coverage. Yes, they said, they can cover me even if I'm overweight, but it's gonna cost me. Okay, it could be worse. After all, last year Blue Cross denied me because I was overweight (based on their weight chart). The problem is that I will *never* be "normal" based on their weight chart because of my big frame. Hearing an insurance agent say, "We can't insure you because you weigh *too much*" is terribly depressing. I think I went numb. It hurt too much to hear.

But then, we get to the medical questionnaire. I'm checking no, no, no on everything *except* a history of depression. Should I lie? Surely they'll pull my medical records and see that I've been on antidepressants. So I tell the truth. Complete silence. Here we go again. She shows me her little chart that says if my depression is "situational" they *may* cover it. But if it has lasted twelve months or more, uh-ohh . . . the alarm goes off. "Crazy person applying for health insurance!" Keep those overweight, depressed people uninsured and let them die! OK, I'm overreacting, but sometimes this whole medical/pharmaceutical system feels like such a racket. Meanwhile, I had to write a check for $300.00 at the pharmacy.

> **"**
> Hearing an insurance agent say, "We can't insure you because you weigh *too much*" is terribly depressing. I think I went numb. It hurt too much to hear.
> **"**

Week 8—Journal Entry #27

Hi Michael,

My gynecologist appointment went well (as well as any gynecologist appointment can go). To my surprise, I had been in 1999 and I didn't even remember! There was nothing out of the ordinary. They want to get the pap results and blood test results from my primary care doctor. And I am due for another mammogram.

One of the things I'm concerned about is that taking Wellbutrin may affect my sleep, which is already not so good. Today will be the first day that I increase the dose, so we'll see what happens.

Today, Lenny is home sick. I'm trying to figure out how I can work out. By the way, I'm now down 7 pounds!

Note to Reader

At this point, L'Tanya had been on Wellbutrin for a couple of weeks. She'd also been using her light box every day with good results. Bear in mind that prior to this, she struggled to stay on course. She was feeling extremely scattered, unmotivated, and overwhelmed. As you read the following entries, see if you notice a "different voice"—one that is far more confident, centered, focused, and full of hope. You'll see that the key to her progress was addressing her UFOs.

Week 8—Journal Entry #28

Hi Michael,
Thanks for checking in. I'm doing great, in good spirits, and being kind to myself. It feels good! I'll send you a journal entry tonight.

Week 9—Journal Entry #29

Whew! I have spent the last three days in a state of panic. I wasn't able to connect to the Internet! I spent thirty minutes on hold waiting for Mindspring tech support, and then another forty-five minutes talking with the tech support guy. We still couldn't get the problem solved.

What I noticed was that this situation made me want to eat. So I did. I didn't empty the fridge, but I was well aware of the fact that my anxiety was the cause. Why eat? Why not do something else (like take a bath or something)? Why do people eat for comfort when there are so many healthier options? I guess that's the million-dollar question.

Although Lenny was sick last week, I still worked out *three times*. I even got up on Saturday morning to go to the gym! Wow. It was nice because the gym wasn't crowded and there were some really good-looking guys there (good eye candy while I walked on the treadmill!). My mother said that Lenny could stay with her for about thirty minutes, so that was a huge help.

No one really knows the kind of stress I have at home, excluding taking care of my mother. For the past five years, I am all Lenny has had. He is so attached to me and is afraid of everything. I can't go anywhere in the house without him. At night, I have to lie down with him to get him to go to sleep. And the lamp has to be on. And I have to hold him. Once he falls asleep, I'll get up and slip out of his room. Last night, he fell asleep and I got up to use the bathroom. I flushed and he woke up. Back in the bed I go. I hear parents talk about letting their child cry, or whatever, until they get tired of it and eventually stop. With Lenny, this doesn't work. So neither of us gets enough sleep.

I often get angry with myself because I think it's my fault—that I created his problem. He spends so much time fighting with me (and trying to manipulate me) that it really wears me out.

I don't like what I see in Lenny and I'm blaming myself for it. But in the past, every time I would beat myself up, it would be followed by some sort of destructive behavior, like overeating. The fact that I haven't been doing this lately is huge for me.

Week 10—Journal Entry #30

On Tuesday, my mother called to say that she'd fallen and couldn't get up. She actually crawled to the phone. So yesterday we spent the morning at the doctor's office. The doctor thinks she tore some ligaments. She was almost there. She was supposed to go to orientation for cardiac rehab on Tuesday. But her leg just gave out. All I could think of was the *Jaws* theme and the line, "Just when you thought it was safe to go back in the water . . . !" I want to scream! I may just do that, but what I'm also going to do is get some support.

Yesterday Ma told me that I was all she had. My mouth opened and some strange voice came out that said, "No, I'm not all you have. There are other people who can help you, but you won't call anyone else." Who said that? Then I asked her to get the names and phone numbers of five people she could call if she needed help because I wouldn't always be able to be "on call," and besides, it's the smart thing to do.

In spite of it all, I'm happy. I don't remember saying that—ever! I don't know . . . maybe it's the medicine "rewiring" my brain? I don't care what it is. For the first time in my life, I can separate my circumstances from who I am. Hell, my circumstances are enough to

> **"** Why eat? Why not do something else (like take a bath or something)? Why do people eat for comfort when there are so many healthier options? I guess that's the million-dollar question. **"**

make anyone want to jump off a building! But I don't want to, thank God. I used to think that I'd be happy if . . . I was involved in a relationship . . . if Jupiter aligned with Mars and peace would guide the planet . . . whatever. It seems kind of funny now.

It reminds me of a passage in the Bible. Jesus is standing in the middle of the ocean, and He's telling someone to walk toward him (or something like that). Whoever it was said, "I can't—I'm afraid." Jesus said look at me—have faith and let go of your fear. That's kind of how I feel. There's this big storm around me (testing me?) and I just have to keep walking straight across the water. I'm gonna get fit. I'm gonna write my book. I'm gonna develop my practice. I'm gonna get remarried. I'm gonna have another baby. And I'm gonna raise a healthy, empowered little boy.

I'm beginning to stand on my own two feet. I'm not defining myself by my circumstances or by whoever is in my life at the time. I finally have faith in myself.

Week 10—Journal Entry #31

Lately I've been inspired to "de-clutter" my house. I'm actually throwing things out! This is a big step for me. Since I started using the light box (and taking Wellbutrin), I'm seeing things with new eyes. I'm finally making some headway, whether it be getting to the gym more often or taking care of things that I've put off for years. It used to be so frustrating the way I would start and stop, start and stop. Now, as I become increasingly more focused (and continue to lose weight), my confidence is improving as well as my self-esteem.

Once a month, my friend Jayne and I are hosting a "ladies night." Last time we went bowling, which was great fun. Fun! I'm having fun! Can you believe it? What a concept!

I've decided to put my classes on hold for the summer. I need time to focus on improving my health and growing my coaching practice. Because when this project is over, I'm determined not to regress.

I've been really busy lately, but amazingly, not overwhelmed (yes, the medication is working!). And like Cheryl suggested, I've been making "absolute yes" lists. This, like so many other things, would not have been possible just a few months ago.

I'm still putting a little pressure on myself to "get everything right," but not nearly as much as in the past. I notice that when I do, it drains my energy. Things really *are* getting better! I thank God for that!

Week 11—Journal Entry #32

Cheryl gave me an assignment to call Michael three times this week to ask for help and/or get encouragement. It was hard. I did call once and it was helpful. But that was it—I was afraid to call again. I've always had this belief that I should only ask for help when I have a *really big* problem! Only then would "bothering" someone be justified.

Hmmm . . . I didn't realize that I felt that way. All I knew was that I didn't ask for help. Very interesting. I'll have to work on that.

I contacted a local TOPS (Take Off Pounds Sensibly) group and I'm going to attend one of their meetings next week. Michael suggested attending a few different meetings (and groups), both to see what is available to me and to get a feel for what would serve me best.

I've been more concerned lately about not getting enough good sleep. It's just like Michael said . . . all of my UFOs are standing in line, waiting patiently to be addressed, and won't stop trying to get my attention until I've dealt with all of them. It's like as soon as I conquer one, the next one in line starts yelling "Hey, look at me, it's my turn!"

So I've not been sleeping well, in large part because of Lenny's schedule. I've been working hard to make his room less cluttered and more inviting so he'll be more comfortable in it (I am so tired of going to bed at 1 or 2 A.M.). Now I'm able to see how much crap he has. No child needs that many toys, especially when all he ends up playing with is a shoebox and a Spiderman with one leg. I've already made one trip to Goodwill and I'm going again this week.

Week 12—Journal Entry #33

My photo shoot is this weekend. I am nervous, of course. As much as I know that I've come a long way, I can't help but measure my success by the pound. You'd think that I would know better. But, you know, it's a process.

I'm afraid that the people who'll be reading this book are going to be as judgmental about me as I am about *myself*—that

L'TANYA

Weight, girth measurements, and body fat percentage, after 12 weeks*:

Height: 5'5"
Weight: 238 lbs. (−12 lbs.)
Chest (bust): 47½" (−2¾")
Waist: 41" (−2")
Hips: 48" (−2½")
Upper thighs: 28¾" (L), 29½" (R) (−2", −2")
Calves: 17¼" (L), 17½" (R) (−½", −½")
Ankles: 9" (L), 9¼" (R) (−¼", −¼")
Upper arms: 15¼" (L), 15¼" (R) (−¾", −¾")
Forearms: 12¾" (L), 13" (R) (−¼", −¼")
Wrists: 7" (L), 7" (R) (−¼", −¼")
Total inches lost: 15¼"
Body fat: 37% (−6%)

*Six weeks of training and dieting.

they won't really care about the fact that I've improved my *life* in so many critical ways. I'm afraid that they'll have a superficial view of the process—that regardless of what I've achieved, all they'll be interested in is how much weight I've lost. I hope there will be people who'll identify with what I've learned, benefit from my experience, and see that they shouldn't lose hope, no matter what challenges they may face.

Note to Reader
At the end of this project, L'Tanya got engaged! If you look at her first journal entries, you'll see how much things can change in twelve weeks!

CHAPTER ELEVEN

BOB

My waist is 38 inches, but I still wear size 34 pants.

Bob

    Age: 33
    Height: 5'9"
    Weight: 211 lbs.
    Occupation: Systems Analyst

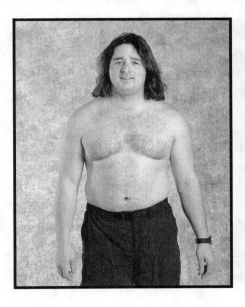 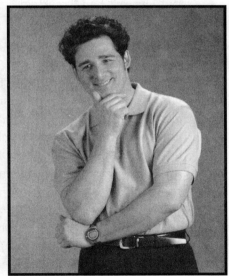

Excerpt from letter:

When I do exercise, I usually start to feel better within a few days. Then I vow to never be out of shape or unhealthy again. But then, for a reason I'm not aware of, I always stop working out. The more that this happens, the harder it is to believe that I'll ever succeed.

Journal Entry #1

Michael,

Thank you for this great opportunity! Now that I'm officially "on board," I actually feel a little nervous. I have to remind myself that as long as I stay focused and give it my all, I'll be fine. Boy, am I excited! I really need to read your book (*When Working Out Isn't Working Out*) because right now, I'm clueless about what this will involve. Regardless, I'm looking forward to getting started!

Journal Entry #2

This morning I had two Dunkin' Donuts (one apple, one jelly). I had a few Munchkins, too. It was at Moynihan Lumber in Beverly (every Saturday they have free donuts and bagels!). Then at Stop and Shop I had half of a Mrs. Fields cookie and a few slices of cheese. But I haven't had "breakfast" yet, so consequently, I am starved.

Journal Entry #3

Well, here I am again (post lunch and dinner). For lunch, I had two burritos, an enchilada, and a small bowl of nachos (covered with globs of fake cheese). I also had some ginger ale. For dinner I had a pork chop, rice pilaf, a salad, and a biscuit. Unfortunately, I couldn't finish my biscuit because it exploded into a million pieces. Now it's after 10:00 P.M. I just finished a large roast beef sandwich. I had some onion rings, too.

Believe it or not, this is typical. I eat like a wild animal. If there's any food around, anywhere, I will eat it. But I don't like to prepare food (I don't have the patience), so I often order takeout or eat on the run. I suppose this will have to change . . .

Journal Entry #4

Last night we went to a Mexican restaurant. It was a lot of fun and very festive. I had some jalapeños stuffed with cream cheese, nachos with salsa, and a chimichanga. I also had two beers and half a margarita.

Today a woman I know asked about my participation in the project. "Why are you doing this?" she asked. "You don't seem to care how you look!" But she's wrong. It's not so much that I'm concerned about what *others* think, it's more about what I think. I'm doing this for *myself*.

Hey, I just had a great idea. I have to go to Moynihan Lumber again. Today I will attempt to forego the complementary donuts! To ensure that I commit to this, I will send this E-mail to you now (before I leave). If I'm successful, it will be a first! But will it be a last?

Journal Entry #5

As a follow-up, I made it past the donut table. But it was much more difficult than I imagined. Those donuts were calling my name. Even now (eight hours later), they are all I can think of. Maybe I'll order a pizza. It will be the sixth time I've had it this week!

Journal Entry #6

Efficiency. That's the name of my game. To me, being efficient means doing as many things as possible at one time. Very rarely am I doing just one thing only. Multitasking is my mantra. For example, I often make calls from my car or while I'm preparing for another task.

I don't like to sleep because it's a waste of time (if I'm asleep, I can't get anything done!). I wake as early as possible and stay up as late as I can. In fact, I often wake up in places where I didn't intend to fall asleep, i.e., slumped over a project or face down in front of my computer. A few days ago, after midnight, I nodded off while completing a project (outside of my house). My only concern was that I was going to pass out cold in my driveway at 1:00 in the morning and freeze to death—an inefficient way to die.

When I commute, I think a lot about how much time is wasted traveling to work and back. On many occasions, I've stayed at work all night. Right now, it's 4:00 and I haven't had lunch yet. Since I'm not tired or lightheaded, I don't think I need to. I refuse to take time to eat when it isn't necessary!

I just finished taking a Palm Pilot "productivity" class, and the teacher was amazing. He was so organized! I would like to be like that someday. What do you think?

> "
> Right now, it's 4:00 and I haven't had lunch yet. Since I'm not tired or light-headed, I don't think I need to. I refuse to take time to eat when it isn't necessary!
> "

Reply from Michael

Hi Bob,

I think you have ADD. And I think we better address it before one of us loses his mind!

I hate using labels for anything, but sometimes there is no other choice. It would be easy to say that you're "easily distracted" or that you have a "concentration problem," but oftentimes, in order to treat this effectively, a doctor has to make a specific diagnosis. This is so he or she can prescribe medication (if necessary) and so your treatment can be covered by insurance.

We will talk more about this. Take the UFO test first. Then I will advise.

Journal Entry #7

I took the quiz you sent me (to assess ADD) and I scored a 28 (out of 30). I was diagnosed with ADD about five years ago. I have also read the book *Driven to Distraction* by Dr. Hallowell, and there is no question that I have this problem.

A few years ago (after I read Dr. Hallowell's book), I went to see my doctor about it and he prescribed Ritalin. Once I started taking it, I was able to study all day with no problem at all. I was also working out daily, losing weight, and feeling great. Ritalin helped me in many ways, but I thought it was "cheating" so I stopped. It definitely helped me to focus, but I felt uncomfortable about the way it seemed to change my personality. When I stopped taking it, I went back to my old ways and, of course, stopped working out.

Journal Entry #8

I'm on my way home from work. Mag is driving. Usually I drive, but I thought this would be a good opportunity to write a journal entry, i.e., an efficient use of my time.

I wanted to touch on some topics that are characteristic of Bob.

I am my own person, unaffected by trends, suggestions, or opinions. Autonomous. I've always been fiercely independent, and rarely do I feel the need to fit in. I'm a nonconformist. A thumbs-up from "Board of Bob" is the only approval I need.

BOB'S UFOs

Attention Deficit Disorder (ADD)
Work Addiction
Poor Life/Time Management
"Askaphobia" (Fear of Asking for Help)
Sleep Apnea
Undertraining
Snack Amnesia
Diet Misconceptions
Weak Boundaries
Self-Sabotage

I am logical. My work is about troubleshooting network and computer problems. This is easy for me and I am good at it. Being logical also keeps me from doing "extraneous" nonproductive things. Like, for example, watching TV, seeing movies, or reading books. Years ago, I started reading novels, but in my mind, they all seemed to run together. I was always getting mixed up with regard to characters, plot lines, etc. So I stopped reading for "pleasure." Besides, it wasn't "productive" compared to other things.

My style of dress is known as "Bobby-Chic." My clothes are comfortable and functional. And since I don't care what others think, they never go out of style. What would I be saying if I bought new clothes all the time, replacing perfectly good clothes that I "thought" I liked? I have clothes that are perfectly fine for wearing around the house, special events, and work. And because I'm so good at choosing them, they can do double, triple, or even quadruple duty!

Just some manifested thoughts . . .

Journal Entry #9

From Mag (Bob's wife)

Dear Michael,
I can't help but put in my two cents about Bob's wardrobe. If you want to know in plain English what Bob means by "Bobby-Chic," it's that he wears only jeans, T-shirts, and sandals all year long (unless

> " My style of dress is known as "Bobby-Chic." My clothes are comfortable and functional. And since I don't care what others think, they never go out of style. "

it's really cold, in which case he'll wear sneakers). For a special occasion, he'll wear a sweater, but it's usually one of mine! Going to weddings is always stressful because I have no idea what the heck he plans on wearing! Sometimes, when cleaning, I will "sacrifice" one of his T-shirts without telling him. It feels good!

When I told our friends that Bob had to bring four outfits to his photo session, everyone laughed and laughed. This is because it'll probably be four pairs of jeans and four different T-shirts! Good luck to your image consultant! Some of his T-shirts are more than ten years old and he refuses to throw them away! I would *love* to see Bob diversify this area of his life!

Reply from Michael

Hi Mag,
Don't worry! He's not fooling anyone! We'll get him straightened out soon enough. But first things first. Before we attend to Bob's image concerns, we have other things to address. While it's true that changing the way Bob looks is one of our primary goals, first we must help him to change how he feels—about both himself and his life! Wait and see what happens! I think you'll be very surprised!

Journal Entry #10

Today I would like to write about something that I think may relate to how I feel about working out.

I have always had problems with being part of a team. I've never liked depending on others, nor have I liked having others depend on me. I really don't like to be told what to do. In high school, I played football for four years. Each one was going to be my last.

Those football practices (particularly during the preseason) were brutal! Four practices a day for an entire week! If someone didn't drop from exhaustion and vomit all over the inside of his helmet, it meant we weren't working hard enough. Ever since, this experience has affected how I feel about exercise. If I *do* go to the gym, I won't let myself leave until I'm sweating buckets and can't feel my arms or legs. Otherwise, I feel like I've wasted my time. I thought I should bring this up . . .

Journal Entry #11

Today I had a physical. All is fine. My weight is the only area of concern (I weigh 211 pounds). I am still digesting that information, along with a bagel, a donut, three cheeseburgers, and half a large pizza. I thought I was around 205, but I guess I was wrong.

Tomorrow I am meeting you (Michael) to discuss my program. I've been looking forward to this for weeks! Winnie the Pooh meets Charles Atlas! See you soon.

Week 1—Journal Entry #12

Today is my first day "on the program." I'm actually a little panicked, especially about the changes you suggested regarding my diet. I'm already afraid that I'm not doing it right, and questioning everything I put into my mouth. I guess this will be a learning process.

I called the YMCA in Beverly and they said that it was okay to work with a trainer who isn't an employee. They also have a nice day care center for Summer (my daughter) that is open until 8:00 P.M. I'll be working out for the first time tonight, so I'll let you know how I do!

❝
Today I had a physical. All is fine. My weight is the only area of concern (I weigh 211 pounds). I am still digesting that information, along with a bagel, a donut, three cheeseburgers, and half a large pizza.
❞

BOB

Weight, girth measurements, and body fat percentage, before:

Height: 5'9"
Weight: 211 lbs.
Chest: 44⅝"
Waist: 38¾"
Hips: 42"
Upper thighs: 23¾" (L), 23¾" (R)
Calves: 16¾" (L), 16⅛" (R)
Ankles: 9¼" (L), 9¼" (R)
Upper arms: 14¼" (L), 14½" (R)
Forearms: 12" (L), 12" (R)
Wrists: 7½" (L), 7¼" (R)
Body fat: 27%

Week 1—Journal Entry #13

Now that I'm "policing" myself, all I can think about is food. I've been studying the diet you gave me. I think this is going to be harder than I thought.

For lunch I went to Stop and Shop. Almost every day I would go there to get a calzone or two slices of pizza. Now I go to the salad bar. So many choices! Today's salad consisted of lettuce, spinach, a sprinkling of carrots, a few cherry tomatoes, broccoli, cucumber, croutons, and a few pieces of grilled chicken (for protein). I doused it with fat-free Italian dressing, grabbed three navel oranges, and headed back to my office. Now I'm going to the water cooler to top off my stomach.

I've been worrying a lot about whether I'm doing this (the diet) right. I suppose that keeping a food log will help.

P.S. I spit out a piece of hard candy that I almost ate by mistake.

Week 1—Journal Entry #14

My first workout was harder than I thought it would be. Not so much physically but mentally. Besides struggling with my technique, I was constantly falling out of line (many of the machines that you want me to use are part of a circuit). Whenever I stretched (between exercises), someone would get on the machine I wanted to use, and I'd have to wait until they were done. I also had a hard time timing my reps. I suppose this will get easier over time.

Week 2—Journal Entry #15

I'm starting to feel more comfortable with my diet. Today's breakfast was something I made myself (according to the plan) and it was actually pretty good! I think Mag and Summer are going to benefit from this (healthy eating) as well.

Today's workout was much better. I'm not as sore, either. I think I'm getting the hang of moving slowly and fluidly and no longer feel the need to time the lift (by counting the seconds it takes to lift and lower the weight). I also worked out on the stationary bike for twenty-five minutes at level five. For a warm-up, I ran around the gym shooting hoops. And you were right—the gym is much less busy at night (8:30–10:00 P.M.). I didn't have any trouble accessing the machines. I also found other machines to use that are not part of a circuit.

Week 3—Journal Entry #16

From Mag (Bob's wife)

Hi Michael,

How are you? Bob and I have been cooking a lot more since he started this project, which is a *rarity*, believe me! (Our neighbors have been joking that the local pizza shop is going to go out of business.)

By the way, can you recommend a cookbook that doesn't require any strange ingredients we've never heard of that we'd have to travel to a specialty shop in the middle of Guatemala to purchase? I think this would really help!

One more thing . . . we have this huge mirror in our bedroom about 6 feet tall and 4 feet wide. Before Bob went to bed last night he stood in front of it for at least ten minutes flexing and admiring his body (I'm not sure he's ever looked in a mirror before!). Anyway, he really enjoyed the time you spent with him in the gym last night and feels really good about what he's doing. Thanks so much for your help!

Week 3—Journal Entry #17

I enjoyed the teleconference—I thought it was a lot of fun. I must say that I think Cheryl was awesome. Rarely am I impressed by anyone, but in this case, I was totally blown away. I could identify with many of the things she said. All day I've been thinking about my homework assignment (making a "statement of intention"). More later!

Week 3—Journal Entry #18

Hola amigo,
I've been to the gym several times since the day you coached me last week, and I'm making good progress.

This weekend I bought a pair of new sneakers. I went to the New Balance outlet and picked out some super-comfy ones. And I actually found a pair that was the right width (I'm an 11½–12 EE or EEEE!). When I think about it, my shoes have always been too small. So every time I would run, my feet felt like they were being folded in half. Maybe I'll enjoy it more now that I won't be in so much pain?

Week 3—Journal Entry #19

I just got back from the gym. My workout was great. But I don't think I'm losing any weight. Every time I step on a scale, I weigh the same. But I do *feel* better, and I think I look better, too. I'm really not too worried, but thought I should let you know.

Week 4—Journal Entry #20

I've been doing well on my diet for two weeks now, and I think it's finally getting easier. This is despite the fact that there's always tons of junk food at work. Today was no different. I was talking to some coworkers when one of them opened a huge bag of Sweet Escapes. Of course, when they were offered to me, I politely declined. I just said, "No, thank you." Nothing more. In my mind I said, "I will *not* allow my success to be compromised by a stupid piece of candy!" The woman who was holding the bag explained that it was low fat (thus, in keeping with my diet). Uh-huh. When I declined (the second time), everyone got quiet. They could tell that I was serious. Serious about my new way of life. It actually felt pretty good!

Week 4—Journal Entry #21

I worked out on Saturday, but it was the first time since week 1 that I felt indifferent about going to the gym. While I was there, it was so hard to stay in the game (mentally). I pushed myself as hard as I could, but I felt like I was going through the motions. I just didn't want to be there. But I stayed and it wasn't until the last ten minutes that I was actually in the mood to exercise.

Over the course of the past two days I ate three brownies and skipped a lot of meals. I knew that I shouldn't have, but I just didn't care. Why?

On a lighter note, my folks came to visit today, which provided me with an opportunity to display my new muscles! My legs have been feeling particularly strong, so I showed them off first. Thursday night my neighbor asked how things were going, so I let her feel me, too. She was clearly impressed! There's no absence of positive feedback here—I feel like a million bucks!

Week 5—Journal Entry #22

People at work are starting to take notice. They're asking me all kinds of questions about what I'm eating and how I'm working out. It's like I'm a walking billboard for this program! My friends are telling me that they see a big difference, too (I tell them all to buy the book).

I tried the interval training that you suggested, and it was fun. I like it because it provides variety—something I really need.

I'm scheduled to see my doctor (regarding treatment for ADD this week). I'll keep you posted.

Week 6—Journal Entry #23

CANDY FOR SALE!
COST: $1.00
KIT KAT, HERSHEY'S, CARMELLO, REESE'S
SPREAD THE WORD, IT'S FOR A GOOD CAUSE!!!

This is the kind of thing that goes on every day around here. Today the candy is sitting right outside my cube. I am being tested . . . again . . .

Week 6—Journal Entry #24

Today I went to see my doctor about ADD. He prescribed Ritalin, the same drug I took once before. Believe it or not, I can already feel a big difference! I think I accomplished more today than I have in the

"

At lunch I ran for
7 miles in the snow
and the rain. It felt
good! It's hard to
believe that only
seven weeks ago, I
was winded going up
one flight of stairs!
Yesterday I ran for
5½ miles and Sunday
I ran 5.

"

past several months! My energy level seems to have increased, too. It seems so strange to be able to focus! I'm excited to see how this affects me over time.

I have a few more appointments set up with my doctor (so, if necessary, he can adjust the timing and dose). Stay tuned.

Week 7—Journal Entry #25

At lunch I ran for 7 miles in the snow and the rain. It felt good! It's hard to believe that only seven weeks ago, I was winded going up one flight of stairs! Yesterday I ran for 5½ miles and Sunday I ran 5.

I have no idea what I weigh now. I don't step on the scale much anymore, but I'm getting smaller. My clothes are now very loose, and my coworkers are still complimenting me on my appearance. I have to admit that getting all this attention is good for my ego, which is a curious thing since, as you know, "I don't really care what anyone thinks."

Week 8—Journal Entry #26

Merrimack River Trail Race (10 Miles), Andover, MA

When I woke up today, I could hardly believe that I was going to run a 10-mile race. Boy, have I come a long way! The race was a lot of fun. The first 3 miles were along the river and the next 4 were up and down some very steep hills (and through streams). When I reached the 8-mile mark, I knew I'd be able to finish without any problem, so I stepped up the pace and ran a little faster. When I came out of the woods, I saw Summer and Mag waiting for me. Summer ran out to meet me just a few feet after I crossed the finish line. What a great moment that was!

Week 9—Journal Entry #27

Do you remember a few weeks ago when I told you that I was losing interest in the project? Now I can't imagine that I ever felt that way. I don't know if it's the Ritalin or just the way I happen to feel today, but whatever the case, I'm relieved. I was so worried that I was going to finish the program and go back to my former ways. Now I'm confident that this won't happen.

From Mag (Bob's wife)

Hi Michael,

Bob is looking good! Everything looks slimmer—his face, his legs, his stomach, his arms—everything! All of his pants are so baggy that it's hysterical! Sometimes when he puts them on, they fall right down to his knees!

I am so happy for Bob—I think he is finally happy with *himself*. Now every time he comes home from the gym he enjoys spending time in front of the mirror (he is a flexing machine!). It is very funny! Good luck with the final weeks of the program!

Week 11—Journal Entry #29

What a great class we had today. I really enjoyed Debbie Ford. I was stunned by what she identified to be my "story," and I've been thinking about it ever since. My story is that I don't care what others think of me, especially with regard to how I look. When she asked me to go back to the time that the story originated, I remembered being nineteen years old. The person I was involved with at the time decided to end our relationship. I was devastated. From that point on, I decided that I didn't care what anyone thought of me. I was protecting myself from being hurt by anyone else. She was right! I do care about how I look! Otherwise, why would I be involved in this project?

Tonight I had a really good workout. It isn't so hard anymore, and I don't know why (could it be because I've been treated for ADD?). I'm not resisting it like I once was. I can finally accept all the time and effort that goes into it.

Tomorrow I'm scheduled to have my image consultation with Ginger. Summer thinks that the color analysis will reveal a strong affinity for pink.

Week 12—Journal Entry #30

I met with Ginger today and it went well. I haven't tried on new clothes in a while (several years!), and guess what—I bought some pants that have a 33-inch waist! *Thirty-three!* When I started the program, my waist was over 38! This is so strange! Seeing myself

> 66
>
> Tonight I had a really good workout. It isn't so hard anymore, and I don't know why (could it be because I've been treated for ADD?). I'm not resisting it like I once was. I can finally accept all the time and effort that goes into it.
>
> 99

BOB

Weight, girth measurements, and body fat percentage, after 12 weeks:

Height: 5'9"
Weight: 181 lbs. (−30 lbs.)
Chest: 41½" (−3⅛")
Waist: 34¼" (−4½")
Hips: 38½" (−3½")
Upper thighs: 23" (L), 22¾" (R) (−¾", −1")
Calves: 15½" (L), 15½" (R) (−¾", −⅝")
Ankles: 9" (L), 9" (R) (−¼", −¼")
Upper arms: 13¾" (L), 13¾" (R) (−½", −¾")
Forearms: 11½" (L), 11½" (R) (−½", −½")
Wrists: 7¼" (L), 7" (R) (−¼", −¼")
Total inches lost: 17½"
Body fat: 15% (−12%)

wearing new clothes is strange as well. I actually look pretty good! I can't remember the last time I thought that.

I feel great. I've decided to continue with the program. I don't want to return to my old bad habits. I'm enjoying this way too much!

My coworkers can't believe my new haircut. They love it. Summer keeps telling me how much she likes it, too. This is the best endorsement for me.

Week 12—Journal Entry #31

Dear Friends,
I am done. Today was my photo shoot.

Twelve weeks ago, I weighed 211 pounds. My body fat was 27 percent. Today I weigh 181 pounds and my body fat is 15 percent. I learned what to eat (and avoid), how to exercise correctly, and how to make lifestyle changes to improve my mental and physical health. I addressed my UFOs (unidentified fitness obstacles) and went from being winded at the slightest bit of exertion to running a 10-mile road race with energy to spare. An image consultant helped me choose new clothes in the right color, style, and size, and I got an "English Wedge" haircut that took ten years off my age. I had an opportunity to be coached by top-notch professionals about topics that ranged from controlling my sweet tooth (Tracy Gaudet, M.D.) to events that altered my psyche more than ten years ago (Debbie Ford). To say the least, this was quite an experience.

Today, a healthy diet and exercise program are an important part of my daily routine. Now I actually *look forward* to working out! (Before, I could hardly stand the thought!) Over the next few months, I'm going to start running road and trail races as an adjunct to my exercise regimen. Participating in this project has been great fun and I've learned *a lot*. It has changed my life *for life*.

CHAPTER TWELVE

JENNIFER

I feel like I'm the fatty, in a sea of slender friends!

Jennifer
Age: 32
Height: 5'½"
Weight: 152 lbs.
Occupation: Pharmaceutical Sales Rep

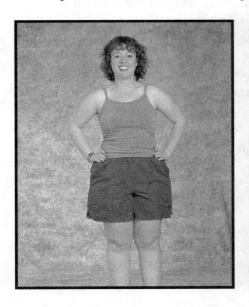 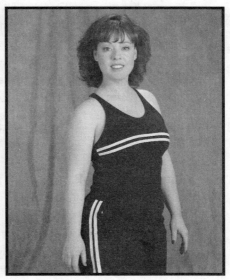

Excerpt from letter:
It seems like every day I'm wishing something: I wish I were 40 pounds lighter. I wish I had more energy. I wish I had the guts to pursue my dreams. It's like I have this huge buffet of opportunities but can't even reach my arm out to spoon any of them on my plate!

Special Considerations

Hashimoto's Thyroiditis (an autoimmune response to proteins in the thyroid gland). This can often cause weight gain, adrenal dysfunction, and chronic fatigue.

Journal Entry #1

Michael,

I'm so excited about this project! Thank you for the opportunity!

Fantasizing about "the new me" has been a lot of fun. This weekend I was at a swing dancing competition. As I watched the other girls who were there to perform, many questions ran through my mind. For example, when I lose weight, will I look like her? Will I have a flat stomach? Will I have leaner legs? In a way, I feel like a little kid looking forward to Christmas Day! I can't wait to unwrap a new me!

Of course, I have some doubts, too. I mean, I think I've been on every diet there is. I've joined Weight Watchers three or four times, tried Jenny Craig, chugged Slim-Fast, been on numerous low-carb plans, been to see a nutritionist, and even did the Fen-Phen thing when it was big several years ago. Every time, it was exactly the same—I'd lose a little weight, start to feel great, and then go off the program. Now, I'm about to have an entire team of experts help me and I'm terrified. Am I going to fail? Do I have the strength to see this through? I'm hopeful, but I'm scared.

Journal Entry #2

This morning I was starving. Like, weak in the knees starving. My stomach was also growling like crazy and I was feeling kind of shaky. By 11:30 A.M. I couldn't wait anymore and had to get some lunch. I was on my way to a sales call, so I went to McDonald's and ordered a Quarter Pounder. I wolfed it down and within an hour or so was feeling fine. But by 4 P.M. my stomach started growling again. How could I be hungry? I had that big burger for lunch?

Believe it or not, this is pretty typical. For example:

- I'm usually very, very hungry by midmorning. I always eat breakfast, but it rarely seems to help.

- My stomach growls and feel crampy (off and on) almost every day.
- Fast food is a regular part of my diet. I'm on the road five days a week (running from one customer to the next), so I often feel like I have no choice. Plus, for me, it's comfort food. I work alone all day, so having a burger (or something at Taco Bell) is like giving myself a treat.
- I rarely eat fruits and vegetables. There just aren't many fruits that I like, and vegetables take too long to cook. I'll order a salad or side of veggies if I'm eating out, but at home it's very rare.

Journal Entry #3

For breakfast today I had Life cereal with 1% milk. By 9:30 A.M. I was starving again. I wonder if I'm not eating enough?

Later in the day I had some time to kill, so I went to say hi to a friend who owns a vintage clothing shop. He had some great dresses he was holding for me, and I quickly tried them on. But while pulling one over my head, I turned to look at my rear view in the mirror. I froze. There were little rolls of fat on my back! *When in the world did I get back fat????* I've always had a big butt and heavy thighs. But back fat??? My God, what next?

Another note: Both yesterday and today (actually, pretty regularly for about a month now), I've had an upset stomach in the afternoon and have had to make a mad rush to find a restroom. My doctor thinks it's stress. I don't think it's related to what I'm eating, because I eat different things all the time.

Reply from Michael

Hi Jenn,
Maybe it is what you're eating? At least in part. Have you ever been tested for candidiasis or irritable bowel syndrome (IBS)? This could go a long way to explain the pattern of fat distribution, weight gain, and other symptoms you describe. What about hypoglycemia? I think that this is all worth looking into. Do you have a doctor who could (would?) run some tests on you? If not, I could recommend someone.

I'm curious to see the results of your UFO test. I don't think that stress can account for everything that's going on with your stomach.

> 66
> *When in the world did I get back fat??? I've always had a big butt and heavy thighs. But back fat??? My God, what next?*
> 99

Journal Entry #4

At exactly 10:30 A.M. (it's like clockwork now), my stomach started growling again.

Later I went to the airport to pick up a friend, but his flight was delayed. While I was waiting my vision started to blur and I felt kind of weak. Once his flight arrived I had something to eat and felt better soon after.

My friends and I spent the evening lounge-hopping. In total, I had three chocolate martinis. By 1 A.M. I was starving, so I had a burger and fries.

Journal Entry #5

Today I curled up on the sofa to read *When Working Out Isn't Working Out*. By the end of the introduction, I was in tears. I could relate to every word on the page! It made me think about all the times I've felt ashamed of my body. For example, once I wore a cropped shirt to a dance club (thinking I looked so good) and overheard a friend say, "Oh great, now we have to look at Jenn's stomach!" And I'll never forget meeting that cute musician who I was chatting with on the phone. After he looked me up and down, he just walked away without saying a word.

This started me thinking . . . Just a few months ago, I was making meals for myself every night. But now, cooking isn't fun anymore. Perhaps the stress I've experienced lately has taken a greater toll than I thought. Within the past three months, my long-term boyfriend broke up with me, my best friend moved across the country to California, I had a cancer scare, and I found out that I was losing my job. That's *a lot of stress!*

Halfway through chapter two of your book, I had another "a-ha" moment. Here's a list of things that would motivate me to work out:

- Walkman (I have one, but I never use it)
- Inspiring musical selections (techno, funk, R&B)

And dance classes! The Dance Complex in Cambridge has hip-hop classes that I've been *dying* to take. But I've always had an excuse (I need the money for other things, it's too far to drive, etc.). Then

> **❝**
> I'll never forget meeting that cute musician who I was chatting with on the phone. After he looked me up and down, he just walked away without saying a word.
> **❞**

JENNIFER'S UFOs

Candidiasis
Hypoglycemia
Food Sensitivities
Seasonal Affective Disorder (SAD)
Irritable Bowel Syndrome (IBS)
Perfectionism
Amino Acid Deficiency
Hypochlorhydria
"Heavy Baggage" Syndrome (Unresolved Emotional Issues)
Adrenal Burnout

I thought about the last class I went to, and how *alive* it made me feel. I was so into it! Heck, that was almost six months ago, and I *still* remember the routine! That's what I need to do, take a new dance class! I made a mental note to get the next class schedule for the Dance Complex and sign up.

I've also been wondering where I should go to do the weight training part of my routine. My apartment complex has a Universal-type gym. What do you think?

Reply from Michael

Hi Jenn,

Regarding a place to work out, I suggest that you explore some other options. It doesn't sound like the gym in your apartment complex has what you're going to need (usually they are very limited in terms of exercise options, and the equipment always needs maintenance). So I would advise rejoining your old health club, or finding another club in your area that has a good atmosphere and full complement of equipment. The dance classes are a good idea, too.

I'd also like you to think (seriously) about preplanning your meals. Do you have a cooler? If not, would you consider buying one? If so, I suggest packing it (every evening) with healthy food choices. This way, you'll have "good" food readily accessible when you get hungry. It may seem like a hassle, but really, what other choice do you have? If you can think of a better idea, I'm all ears!

Random thoughts . . . With regard to what you've told me thus far, I guess step one is to confirm (or rule out) any underlying medical problems that are contributing to your blood sugar swings, hunger, weight gain, etc. The results of your UFO test will give us a good sense of what we need to address first. Step two will be to do some cognitive work around your response to particular types of stress (for example, working with customers and appearing in image-conscious social situations). I'd also like to do some energy work to address your food cravings. Sound good?

Journal Entry #6

So, here's my thought . . . If I can get my big ol' butt going, I'll take dance classes on Thursday and Friday evenings. On the other days, I'll either work out at the gym or go to the aerobics annex. What do you think?

Journal Entry #7

Hi Michael,
I know that we haven't "officially" started yet, but for now, do you have any suggestions about what I should do? Should I just concentrate on getting my big ol' butt moving, no matter what it entails? *grin*

Reply from Michael

Hi Jenn,
Before we go any further, would you please do me, and especially yourself, a big favor? As in not joking anymore about your butt! You see, the problem, Jenn, is that it's at your own expense! You're just being funny, I know, but remember, your body is humor-impaired! As a matter of fact, it totally buys whatever you think and say. So let's stop the self-deprecating comments. Agreed?

Week 1—Journal Entry #8

For lunch today I had a spinach salad with carrots, tomatoes, grilled chicken, and two tablespoons of dressing. It came with a roll. In my mind, all I could hear was "Jeeeeennnnnnnn … you know you want to eat meeeee!" But I didn't.

By the way, why can't you put me on a cheese and chocolate diet? I'm thinking it would be easier to stick to. What do you think?

Actually, you'll be pleased to hear that since starting the plan (for candidiasis), I've had more energy, my head has been clearer, and my stomach has calmed down. For the first few days, though, I felt a little achy and tired. Is this normal?

Reply from Michael

When you stop "feeding" candida (by not eating foods that contain yeast), you may initially feel a little sick (achy, feverish, tired). This is due to the yeast "dying off" in your body and is only temporary. The good news is that if you've been feeling this way, it's just more confirmation that we're on the right track with regard to your problem. The fact that your head felt clearer and your blood sugar seemed more stable is a good sign, too.

Week 1—Journal Entry #9

I had a date tonight, but he cancelled. Drat! So there I was, all

---

JENNIFER

Weight, girth measurements, and body fat percentage, before:

Height: 5'½"
Weight: 152 lbs.
Chest (bust): 36"
Waist: 31½"
Hips: 44¾"
Upper thighs: 26" (L), 26¾" (R)
Calves: 15¼" (L), 15½" (R)
Ankles: 9" (L), 9" (R)
Upper arms: 11½" (L), 11½" (R)
Forearms: 9¼" (L), 9¼" (R)
Wrists: 5¾" (L), 5¾" (R)
Body fat: 34%

dressed up with nowhere to go, pacing around my apartment, wondering what to do. Should I go to the movies? Stay in? Call a friend? I had three cookies and tossed the rest into the trash.

So I headed to my favorite blues club. I sat at the bar and ordered a decaf coffee and a chilled shot of vodka (vodka is okay once in a while, right?). I also had a diet Coke (can I have diet drinks?).

Question: What can I use for a salad dressing if I can't have vinegar or mayo (on Plan C)?

By the way, aerobic exercise bores me. I see everyone else hauling ass (looking like they're really into it) while I'm counting every second until I'm done. Why am I so different?

And those crunches you showed me hurt! I think it's a good pain, though. (What's that saying, "Pain is weakness leaving the body"?)

Reply from Michael

Hi Jenn,

Regarding abdominal crunches . . . this is a perfect example of why it's important to use strict form. Most people feel that doing eight to twelve reps of this exercise slow feels far more effective than doing fifty (or more) repetitions fast. It sounds like you would agree!

With regard to salad dressings, try olive oil with lemon and spices. If you absolutely can't stomach it, you can add a tiny bit of vinegar. But if it bothers your stomach, don't.

Regarding alcohol, it depends on what "every once in a while" means (and what you mix it with). And what it makes you do!

Regarding diet drinks, by and large, you should stay away from anything containing aspartame, artificial sweeteners, and chemical preservatives. Once or twice a week probably won't kill you—but it won't help you, either.

And last, regarding aerobic exercise: You have to remember that you're just getting started, meaning that it doesn't make sense to compare yourself to other people. Also, once you work through the "break-in" phase you should begin to experience what you're doing as invigorating (as opposed to tedious) and focused (as opposed to dull). Then people will be looking at you thinking "Wow, she's really into it—why am I so different?"

Week 2—Journal Entry #10

Home for the holidays. Stepped on my mom's scale today. 147.8 pounds. I love digital scales! 147.8 looks so much better than 148! Mom says my face looks thinner than when she saw me in the spring. My pants fit a little bit better, too.

Week 2—Journal Entry #11

Merry Christmas. I spent most of the day with my mother and brother, but it wasn't exactly a joyous occasion. First I had to watch my brother eat a whole box of chocolates. Then he gave me a really hard time when I had just one little piece! Later, I had one bite of potato salad and he got on my case again. I lost it. I spent the entire evening crying in my room, feeling like a failure for having one piece of candy on Christmas. Bah, humbug.

Week 2—Journal Entry #12

I decided to go home a day early. My mother wasn't happy about this, and we argued about it. She means well but doesn't always understand where I'm coming from. During dinner, for example, she kept asking me things like, "Are you sure you're allowed to put margarine on that? Does Michael know you eat this?" I know that she's just trying to keep me on track, but I don't like being so closely scrutinized, especially when I'm already feeling vulnerable.

The good news is that I now weigh 146.8, down another pound! And the skirt that I wore home, which I haven't put on in a month, is actually a bit loose now (it used to be skintight!).

Week 3—Journal Entry #13

Lunch was quinoa pasta with tomatoes, garlic, and crabmeat, sautéed in sesame oil. Later I left my apartment to go to the gym, but lo and behold, one of my front tires was flat. I don't think God wants me to exercise!

Week 3—Journal Entry #14

Today I stopped at McDonald's for an egg sandwich (minus the English muffin). What a mistake! Soon after, I was sick to my stomach. Looks like I won't be doing that again!

Week 3—Journal Entry #15

Breakfast was coffee and a protein shake (made from whey protein powder) and a single serving of rice milk I brought from home. At 1 P.M. (while shopping) I suddenly felt very shaky. Luckily there was a Taco Bell nearby, and I ordered two chicken tacos. For the rest of the afternoon I played Dance Dance Revolution until I was ready to drop.

Being away from home is hard. During the day, my coworkers eat a lot of junk food (in particular, burgers and fries) and I can't escape the smell. Then at night, everyone drinks. So much forbidden fruit . . .

On a more positive note, I feel good in the outfit I'm wearing today. My pants used to be skintight! Now they fit perfectly! Woo-hoo!

> **❝**
> Later I left my apartment to go to the gym, but lo and behold, one of my front tires was flat. I don't think God wants me to exercise!
> **❞**

Week 3—Journal Entry #16

Today was a milestone. For the first time in a long time, I actually wore pants *without* a shirt tied around my waist! You could almost say they were loose! Progress!

Week 3—Journal Entry #17

I had a good workout today! I'm getting stronger!

I will admit, though, that I had a few drinks to celebrate the new year. Between 6 P.M. and 5 A.M. (bedtime), I had three glasses of champagne, half a glass of red wine, and a small snifter of cognac. I was proud of myself (because I didn't have that much alcohol), especially considering the circumstances (New Year's party).

> **❝**
> For the first time in a long time, I actually wore pants *without* a shirt tied around my waist! You could almost say they were loose! Progress!
> **❞**

Week 4—Journal Entry #18

I started my new job today!

My weight was up a pound this morning. Should I be worried? I'm now between 144 and 145. Hmmm . . .

I ran into my neighbor today and she asked me if I was losing weight. So I guess it's starting to be noticeable, even after only 8 pounds or so!

Week 4—Journal Entry #19

Today I had to get up at 5:30 A.M. It was hard to get up so early, but I wanted to go to the gym because I'd skipped it the day before. My weight is back down to 143! Thank God!

I had a good workout today. I'm able to do more reps on each machine. And that ab exercise! Wow! I would've never believed that using the "right" technique could make that much of a difference!

Week 5—Journal Entry #20

On the way home from work I stopped to pick up some groceries. I swear, I almost lost it. Walking past the bakery section, I was dying for pastry (and I'm not even a big pastry person). When I passed the dairy section, I fantasized about downing a gallon of egg nog. Ramen noodles, sugary cereal . . . you name it, I wanted it. I guess it's the whole "forbidden fruit" thing (you want what you can't have). Does this ever go away?

Week 5—Journal Entry #21

I'm a little disappointed in myself. I didn't lift weights today. I walked, and it was good exercise, but I missed going to the gym. I'll do better next week.

Week 5—Journal Entry #22

My weight is down another pound! I now weigh 142! I did a little happy dance around my apartment.

Victory of the day: tucking in my shirt!

Week 5—Journal Entry #23

For some reason, for the past week or so, I've been feeling really inadequate—like I should've lost more weight than I have. Granted, a little over a month ago I was 152 pounds. Now I'm down to 141, which is encouraging. But I'm afraid that when all is said and done, people won't be able to tell that I've lost that much weight. I worry that the other participants are doing much better than I am, and that you'll have to say,

"Jennifer had good intentions but was the one person in our group who failed."

I know that I'm doing pretty well, but I guess I'm feeling a bit insecure. I often gauge my success by how I compare to others. If I'm doing better than everyone else, I rock. If not, I suck.

Anyway, my appointment with Dr. Rothfeld was interesting. He suggested that I could have some "adrenal issues" and that my cortisol level may be raised. He also thinks that testing my urine, blood, and saliva should be our next step.

Later that day, when I arrived for my meeting, everyone had just finished lunch (pizza). I was glad that I had eaten beforehand (so that I wasn't tempted). There were snacks everywhere—M&Ms, 7-layer Mexican dip, home-baked chocolate chip cookies . . . you name it. Later in the afternoon, I had a few handfuls of popcorn and five tortilla chips.

One of my coworkers joked, "Are you going to record that in your journal?" I know he was just joking, but part of me wanted to sock him. So as he bit into his chocolate chip cookie I replied, "Yes, cookie-boy, it's going in my journal!"

After the meeting, I headed to the gym. I had a 6 P.M. appointment with one of the trainers (to make sure that I was positioned correctly on the equipment). It was partly helpful and partly discouraging. The discouraging part was that I had the feeling he thought I was an idiot! Like, how could a girl like me (who isn't a gym bunny in a thong) be featured in a book? He also told me that the workout you gave me is too easy—that I should be doing at least three sets of everything ("Otherwise, what's the point?").

He gave me the impression that I shouldn't even bother if my workout wasn't going to be "hardcore." He also asked why I was trying to isolate individual muscle groups instead of performing a few exercises that would work on many groups at once. I was annoyed that I was being put on the defensive, so I gave him a silent "screw you" and went about my business.

> **"**
> I worry that the other participants are doing much better than I am, and that you'll have to say, "Jennifer had good intentions but was the one person in our group who failed."
> **"**

Hi Jenn,

Just so you know, beating yourself up is not allowed on this program! Comparing yourself to others is also "strictly prohibited." You must learn to trust the process. And to trust yourself (to be doing the right thing, regardless of how anyone else is doing).

Also, regarding your concern about not losing enough weight . . . depending on who you talk to, the optimum rate of weight loss is 1 to 2 pounds a week. If you lose weight any faster than this, you're apt to lose more than just fat (not to mention slowing down your metabolism, which is the last thing you want to do!). So you're right on schedule, Jenn! Good job!

Now about your gym experience . . . try not to let it get you down. I'm sure that your trainer meant well. But it sounds like he has a different way of looking at things. To reiterate:

(a) one of the biggest mistakes people make (when beginning a program) is trying to do too much too soon (Cycle 1 is designed to help you get your feet wet without getting sore, hurting yourself, or getting confused);

(b) I don't believe that you need "at least three sets of an exercise" to achieve optimum gains (if you always move very slowly and do as many strict reps as you can, one or two sets of an exercise will be all that you'll ever need); and

(c) in my experience, to increase muscle tone and contour, isolation movements are far more effective than those that involve several muscle groups at the same time. Feel better now?

Week 6—Journal Entry #24

Whenever I eat anything that has the slightest bit of yeast or wheat, my stomach (and bowels) go haywire! Obviously, cutting these things out is a good thing!

Week 6—Journal Entry #25

I went to the gym on the way home from work. Had a pretty good workout! I can feel myself getting stronger! I swear my upper arms aren't as big and flabby anymore, and my hips look smaller, too! I left the gym feeling energized!

Week 6—Journal Entry #26

Today, as I was rushing to get ready for work, I reached w-a-a-a-y back into my closet and pulled out the suit that I wore for my first Merck interview (almost five years ago). I never wore it again because ever since, it has been too tight. But now, it fits beautifully! Woo-hoo!

Week 6—Journal Entry #27

I now weigh 140 pounds! Yay!

Week 6—Journal Entry #28

Today at lunch I ordered a small salad and chicken parm (without the pasta). I really, *really* wanted the pizza (that everyone else was eating), but I've been cheating too much lately, so I abstained. I have to get back on track.

> 66
>
> Whenever I eat anything that has the slightest bit of yeast or wheat, my stomach (and bowels) go haywire! Obviously, cutting these things out is a good thing!
>
> 99

Week 6—Journal Entry #29

I'm in California visiting my friend Cat. We left her house tonight at 10 to go dancing. I was feeling a bit self-conscious because, well, it's California, and I expected to see nothing but tiny, perfect-looking blondes in sexy, skimpy outfits. But I must have looked okay because a lot of guys asked me to dance. *Plus*, even though there were women there who were in really good shape, there were also women who were heavier than me and/or not as well dressed. Once I realized this, I was able to loosen up and enjoy myself. Cat and I each drank two vanilla vodkas and danced until 1:30 A.M.

Week 6—Journal Entry #30

Clothing victories today:

- I wore a skirt to my meeting today that I haven't worn in a couple of years! I'm fitting into size 10s now!

- Tonight I wore a short-sleeved T-shirt. I wore the same shirt a month ago and had to stretch the sleeves out because they were too tight on my arms. Tonight it fit fine! The program must be working!

Week 6—Journal Entry #31

I think my stomach is more sensitive now to wheat and yeast, because less than thirty minutes after eating a pasta salad, I had to make a run for the bathroom. I was sick to my stomach!

This afternoon they had a cake for one of my coworkers (it was her birthday). I had a slice (to share in the festivities). Around 3:30 P.M. I was hungry again but resisted having any more cake. I had a bite-sized Snickers bar instead. Not good, but better than a slice of cake!

Week 6—Journal Entry #32

Deep Thoughts:

- I wish you could delay the book. I feel like I need more time! The 15 or 20 pounds I'll lose by the end doesn't seem enough. I'd love for people to see what I look like after I've lost 40! A lot of wonderful things have happened thus far—my eating habits have changed (dramatically), my energy level has increased, my stomach almost never bothers me anymore, and I'm down a whole size! But I'm worried that it's not very obvious.
- I feel bad about the way I've been living my life. On Monday (during the teleclass), I listened to Bob and L'Tanya talk about their crazy schedules, kids, ailing mother, demanding job, etc. And then there's me, whining about being bored (surfing the Net and watching TV). I'm sure they would kill to have just five minutes to themselves! I'm ashamed of myself.

Week 6—Journal Entry #33

Our workout this evening was a lot of fun! I'm so glad you came down! I still can't believe that you inspected my fridge! I wasn't prepared for that!

With you putting me through the paces, my workout was very tough! But it was good that you were there, because it showed me that I wasn't working hard enough. For all the joking I did (screaming "I hate you" as you made me move slower or do an extra rep), I was very appreciative!

Week 7—Journal Entry #34

This morning I slept until 8 A.M. Got out of bed and ouch. Yep, my muscles are definitely cursing you!

Tonight I went to a Mexican restaurant. I ordered seafood baked in tomato sauce with steamed veggies on the side. Instead of rice, I asked if I could have beans (as a substitute). This got me thinking . . . I'm sure a lot of people would be hesitant to do this. But if they were allergic to peanuts, for example, wouldn't they let their wait person know about it? So why shouldn't I be the same way with yeast? If yeast makes me feel poorly, I should avoid it. End of story.

Week 7—Journal Entry #35

Up at 6:30 A.M. According to my scale, I now weigh 138! Down another pound!

Week 7—Journal Entry #36

Hi Michael,

I'm in tears right now. I just got word from my manager that our corporate folks have changed their minds . . . I have to go through basic training, which means that I'll be away for the next six weeks!

God, the remainder of my program in a hotel, sitting in lectures all day and studying all night . . . hotel food three meals a day . . .

I'm really going to need your help! I'm afraid that I'll gain all the weight back! What am I going to do?

Week 7—Journal Entry #37

For dinner tonight, John and I went to a new restaurant. I have to admit, Michael, that I did splurge a bit on dinner. Okay, a lot. I had roast pork loin with mashed potatoes and a side of mixed veggies. I also had a vanilla vodka and diet Coke. We also ordered dessert (ice cream cake) and I ate half of it.

I guess in retrospect, I did okay. The old me would have eaten everything and had more than one drink. I can also see that I'm eating to comfort myself—to deal with the stress of being away from home for six weeks. I need to make sure that this doesn't happen while I'm away.

Week 7—Journal Entry #38

Tonight I went dancing. I had a wonderful time! Most of my clothes were packed already, so my clothing selection was limited. In the back of my closet, I found this leopard-print dress that I'd bought two years ago but never worn. It still had the tags on it! The plan was to lose weight (so I could actually wear it), but I eventually gave up. Anyway, for a hoot I tried it on and it looked great! So off I went to the dance, in a "new" leopard-print dress, 15 pounds lighter than the last time my friends saw me! All night, people were asking me if I'd lost weight or done something new. It was wonderful!

Week 7—Journal Entry #39

Spent the whole day with John wandering around Harvard Square (window-shopping and talking). In the afternoon we stopped at our favorite ice cream place and split one scoop of honey-walnut ice cream. Later that evening, he took me to a really nice Italian restaurant for a going-away dinner. I definitely went off the program. I had a roll with some olive oil, a glass of red wine, and a house salad. For dinner I had lobster ravioli with shrimp and scallops. After dinner, we ordered a chocolate mousse cake to split. I can't say that I didn't enjoy it, but I paid for it later on.

Week 7—Journal Entry #40

Well, here I am "in training."

In general, these are my greatest challenges thus far:

- Food, food, everywhere!

> **"**
> God, the remainder of my program in a hotel, sitting in lectures all day and studying all night . . . hotel food three meals a day . . . I'm really going to need your help! I'm afraid that I'll gain all the weight back! What am I going to do?
> **"**

- Lo-o-o-ong lectures all day. We get breaks, but I'm not used to sitting for so long! I feel like I need caffeine or sugar to keep me going.
- Restaurant meals three times a day.
- All the female reps are thin and cute. I often compare myself to them.

Week 8—Journal Entry #41

My workout sucked. The fitness center was packed and the equipment is old and in poor condition. I couldn't even get on a machine. It was like musical chairs (trying to get on one before the next person jumped in). So I finally gave up and left.

Week 8—Journal Entry #42

Today I studied until 10:30 P.M. At 9 P.M. I took a stress break and went a bit nuts. I raided my minibar and ate a bag of cheddar popcorn and some peanut M&Ms. It was everything building up: stress, missing home, being lonely, and cravings (due to PMS). So I just let loose.

Week 8—Journal Entry #43

I had an hour to kill before lunch, so I went to my room to get the key to the minibar. I brought it to the front desk and told them to keep it because I didn't want to be tempted anymore.

I decided to drive home for the weekend. The drive was long, but I was glad to be away from the hotel. I hadn't been outside since I checked in on Sunday! At 6 P.M. I stopped to get something to eat. I went off my program *again* (I had chicken nuggets and fries). Within thirty minutes I was sick to my stomach.

I'm happy to be home for the weekend, but my energy is low, my muscles are in knots, and my stomach (although it doesn't hurt or growl) feels bloated and uncomfortable.

According to my scale, I now weigh 140 (up 2 pounds). Whew! I thought it would be worse, especially with all the crappy food I've been eating. But now I have to start *losing* again! I'm tired of being in maintenance mode!

Week 8—Journal Entry #44

Last night (Saturday) John and I went out to dinner. While waiting
for a table, I started feeling shaky. I broke into a sweat and my
heart started pounding. Then it occurred to me that I hadn't eaten
in almost eight hours!

We asked for some tortilla chips and salsa (I ate half the bas-
ket). I was afraid I would faint if I didn't eat something right away. I
felt stupid for letting this happen. I was so busy running errands
that I forgot to eat!

Week 9—Journal Entry #45

Back to the grindstone (training). I was dragging all morning. I just
couldn't wake up. At lunch, I had a salad, but the evening snack was
hard to resist. They had a huge spread of sweets, including fresh-
baked cookies, carrot cake (my favorite), and chocolate mousse
cake. But somehow I managed to grab a bunch of red grapes and get
the heck out of there before I did any damage.

Week 9—Journal Entry #46

Tonight I went to dinner with some coworkers. I ended up ordering a
drink (a Manhattan) before we ate. Then, after dinner (a burger and
fries), I ordered a second drink but only had a few sips. I went to bed
at 9, and tossed and turned for about an hour.

Week 10—Journal Entry #47

Yay! I'm going home today! Everyone is complaining about their
weight (after three weeks of eating hotel food). Several people have
asked me for the title of your first book. We're all getting pretty
desperate!

Week 10—Journal Entry #48

It is so good to be home!

Dinner was really nice. We went to Figs (one of Todd English's
restaurants). John and I split an appetizer of polenta with wild

> " I had an hour to kill
> before lunch, so I
> went to my room to
> get the key to the
> minibar. I brought it
> to the front desk and
> told them to keep
> it because I didn't
> want to be tempted
> anymore. "

mushrooms. For my entrée I had lamb and veggies. It was rather rich, so I didn't eat the whole thing. I also had a glass of red wine. Fell asleep around 11 P.M.

Week 10—Journal Entry #49

Tonight I went to the mall. I decided to try on a suit, despite the fact that it was a size 10 (I usually take a size 14, or a big 12, in suits). Before I went into the dressing room, I grabbed a few more (all size 10) to see if any would fit.

Michael, *they all fit great!!!!!*

I hadn't bought a suit (with pants) in at least five years, because the pants were always too small. But not this time! I can only imagine how I'll feel when I'm able to wear a size 8!

Week 10—Journal Entry #50

I didn't do well today. This afternoon I had a glass of red wine and a few carby snack things (I was pretty hungry, even before the wine). I also had a pita wedge with hummus, ⅛ of a wheat bagel with cream cheese and lox, and a handful of chips. And of course, I crashed later on. As I was driving John home around 6 P.M., I started to get really shaky. So we stopped at Bertucci's for dinner. I had a roll with a pat of butter while we waited to be seated. For dinner we ordered a pizza. I ate the topping (cheese, onion, and meatball) and left the crust.

Week 10—Journal Entry #51

I had a bowl of cereal for breakfast and a cup of coffee on the way to class. A little while later, my stomach was killing me. I was getting sick every ten minutes or so. I think it might be my new cereal. I started eating it yesterday, and that's when the problem started. Needless to say, I tossed the rest of it in the trash.

This evening (for dinner) we were treated to four-foot-long subs. I had part of one with some salad. The bread started bothering me shortly after, and I felt bloated and gross. By 7 P.M. I was exhausted and my stomach was still upset. I decided to give myself a break and headed back to my room.

Week 11—Journal Entry #52

Last day of training!

    I left after lunch to drive home. Stopped on the way for a cup of coffee and a Krispy Kreme donut (to celebrate). Dinner was six chicken nuggets and a bottle of water.

Week 11—Journal Entry #53

It is so good to be home! Lunch was on the run (a burger with half the bun). Dinner was a chicken sandwich and a handful of fries, which (surprise) made me sick to my stomach. I ate that on the run as well, as I headed into Boston to see John. Around 10 P.M. we went out with some friends to celebrate. I had a few sips of beer and a few tablespoons of hummus with a small wedge of pita bread. Which, of course, upset my stomach. No more bread for me!

Week 11—Journal Entry #54

I think I figured out why I've been so tired this week! The soup I've been eating contains hydrolyzed soy protein (which always knocks me out). They might as well call it "Jennifer's Sleepytime Soup"!

    Time to celebrate! I'm now a debt-free woman! My bonus came in the mail today, and I rushed it to the bank. It's more than I thought it would be—enough to pay off my car loan and my last credit card (and start a savings account). What a huge weight off my shoulders! It feels great to have it all gone!!!

Week 11—Journal Entry #55

Since I've been home I've been making better food choices (better, but not perfect). For instance, Monday I had an all-day business meeting. Lunch was assorted wrap sandwiches, chips, and cookies. I ate an egg salad wrap and had half of an oatmeal cookie. Tuesday night wasn't good, either. John and I went out for dinner, and we were both starving, so he ordered nachos for an appetizer. And of course, I had a few . . .

I haven't gone to the gym this week. I've been running errands, doing work at night, and getting ready for my mom's visit. My gym stuff was packed and sitting in the back seat of my car, but it was hard to justify going with all the work I had to do. But I'm going on Monday, I swear! I'm looking forward to it!

Week 11—Journal Entry #56

Today I had dinner at an Italian restaurant. I had a breadstick and a grilled chicken breast in a mushroom sauce. After dinner, John and I had coffee and split a dessert (bananas broiled with some brown sugar over gelato).

I feel guilty. I haven't gone to the gym in two weeks.

Reply from Michael

Hi Jenn,

I've been looking over your journal entries. Looking back, I think I should have been more assertive about providing you some direction, especially with regard to your eating habits while you were away from home. Don't get me wrong—I'm thrilled that you were able to hold your own under such trying circumstances (no small feat, considering the pressure you were under). But I'm wondering if you may have needed more from me. I was trying to be sensitive to the fact that you were under so much stress, but perhaps this wasn't really in your best interest. Any thoughts?

Week 11—Journal Entry #57

Honestly, Michael, for me, you did the right thing. If you had pressured me in the slightest bit, even in the past week or so since I've been back, I would have cracked. I'm just happy that I held my own. Now I can pick up where I left off five weeks ago.

Note to Reader
It's important to note that Jenn's job was not the sole cause of her weight-loss plateau. Often a new relationship can create diet challenges, too! In fact, oftentimes when people become involved in a new romance, they start to dine

out and drink a lot more, and as a result, gain weight. Consider this food for thought (especially if you're beginning to date!).

Week 12—Journal Entry #58

I had a great workout today! I hadn't realized how much I missed my gym! Overall, I feel much stronger and healthier. Sure, I still have weight to lose. But I can see that I am getting more toned and that I'm much better proportioned than I was when I started. Even though I've been inconsistent, I can see a big change. I can't even imagine how much I would have improved (had I stayed with the program).

Week 12—Journal Entry #59

Well, Michael, the past few months have certainly been an exciting ride. Here are a few of my thoughts regarding what I've learned and achieved:

- I lost 15 pounds, an amazing feat considering what I've been through. Even though for six weeks I had to work and live in a hotel, I didn't gain any weight and managed to exercise twice a week.
- Because of my thyroid problem, I've been about the same weight for years! It wasn't until I addressed my problem with yeast that this all changed.
- I've gone from a size 14 to 10 and can even fit into some 8s!
- For the first time since I left college, I'm completely out of debt.
- I don't watch TV much anymore, which frees up a lot of time. I spend more time getting organized now, which helps me to get more done.
- Even though I'm not perfect, I no longer beat myself up. Now when I cheat, I no longer feel like a failure (and give up).
- I've learned how to do my hair so that it looks better and takes less time!
- I no longer have stomach problems as long as I eat the right foods. Every once in a while if I eat something with sugar or yeast, my stomach growls and gets crampy (but much less than it did before).

JENNIFER

Weight, girth measurements, and body fat percentage, after 12 weeks:

Height: 5'½"
Weight: 137 lbs. (−15 lbs.)
Chest (bust): 35¼" (−¾")
Waist: 29½" (−2")
Hips: 41" (−3¾")
Upper thighs: 24" (L), 24½" (R) (−2", −2¼")
Calves: 14½" (L), 14¾" (R) (−¾", −¾")
Ankles: 8¾" (L), 8¾" (R) (−¼", −¼")
Upper arms: 11" (L), 10¾" (R) (−½", −¾")
Forearms: 9" (L), 9" (R) (−¼", −¼")
Wrists: 5½" (L), 5½" (R) (−¼", −¼")
Total inches lost: 15"
Body fat: 27% (−7%)

- Soon I'll be singing and acting, something I've wanted to do for years. And now I have a new boyfriend to support me each step of the way.
- I have a whole new wardrobe (consisting of clothes that were once too small!).
- Perhaps my greatest accomplishment is that I've made this a way of life. With programs I tried in the past, I'd usually quit within two or three weeks!

Thank you, Michael, for your advice and support for the past twelve weeks. It's hard to believe that with all I've learned, I've only just begun!

CHAPTER THIRTEEN

MANDY

For most of my life I've had low self-esteem—
it's time to give it a boost.

Mandy

Age: 22
Height: 5'3½"
Weight: 182 lbs.
Occupation: Student, psychology (University of South Dakota)

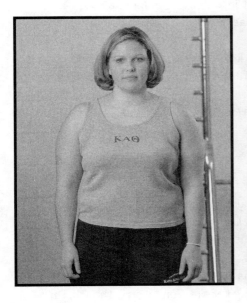 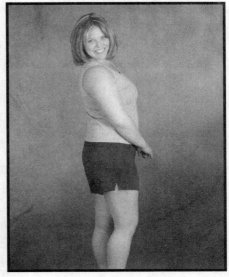

Excerpt from letter:

Soon I'll be graduating from college and going on job interviews (where
first impressions mean everything). I want to be confident about how
I look. Right now, I don't like what I see.

Journal Entry #1

Wow! That was about all I could say when I found out I was chosen.
I know that this won't be easy, but I'm going to give it my best.
I'm very excited about this opportunity. I can't wait to get started!
I can't wait to see the results!

Journal Entry #2

Hi Michael,
I just saw pictures from a recent trip to Las Vegas . . . goodness,
help me! How did I let this happen? Where is the nearest spin class?

Journal Entry #3

Michael,
Okay, you're going to kill me. Might as well kick me out of the
makeover project right now. I get into Boston on Monday at
11:50 P.M.! Ouch! I know—I'm a master when it comes to making
things complicated . . .

　I really apologize. If you would like to call and ream me a good one,
feel free, but hey, I saved $150! That's a lot of money for a college
student!

　Will you forgive this podunk girl from South Dakota?

Journal Entry #4

Hi Michael,
Well two-and-a-half days and counting! I can't wait to begin my
"transformation"! I'm tired of feeling fat and out of control. I hope
that you're as enthusiastic about this as I am! That's a stupid
thought . . . why wouldn't you be?

　I'm afraid to say that I may have strep throat. There are some
lovely puss pockets forming on my tonsils. Don't worry, though, I'm
making the trip, regardless of how I feel. I wouldn't miss this opportunity for anything! Being selected to participate in this project has
been one of the best things that has ever happened to me!

　I've been a little irresponsible lately, especially with regard to
taking care of myself and keeping up with my studies. I think this is

due, in no small part, to my low self-esteem. I'm hoping that this project will help put me on the right track. And what a time to be doing this! New year, new semester, new start! Thank you again for this wonderful opportunity!

Journal Entry #5

Michael,
I'm having some troubling feelings today and I wanted to share them with you.

I'm getting ready to go out to dinner with my friends. As I look in the mirror, all I see is how chubby my face looks and how much weight I've gained. How could I have let myself get this way? Why didn't anyone say anything to me? Actually, my boyfriend has said plenty. Do I dare say he's been right?

My friends say I look fine. I don't know, though. Lately I've been feeling very unattractive. Is it my low self-esteem that makes me overeat? I do know that food gives me instant gratification. And I know that for me, this need for an immediate reward will be a major obstacle.

When I think about getting started, I feel anxious about how I look. What if I'm *too* fat? What if when I meet Michael he says, "Oh no, she didn't look *that* big in her pictures!" The truth is that I need this now more than ever. I'm in such a rut! And getting involved in this project is like calling a tow truck to pull me out of a ditch. I hope that the truck can do it! It's not that I doubt you or the effectiveness of the program—it's just that I feel like an eighteen wheeler (compared to a compact car). How's that for an analogy!

I can tell this is going to be the hardest thing I've ever done. And I'm going to need a lot of support. I don't think I can do it alone.

Journal Entry #6

Hi Michael,
Well, I'm on my way! I guess if there is a plane crash today, and I don't show up, you can assume it was me. Horrible, horrible . . . I know. Don't worry—it won't happen!

I'm very excited to close this current chapter of my life and start a new one. See you soon!

> " As I look in the mirror, all I see is how chubby my face looks and how much weight I've gained. How could I have let myself get this way? Why didn't anyone say anything to me? Actually, my boyfriend has said plenty. Do I dare say he's been right? "

Journal Entry #7

Hi Michael,

My flight and trip home were just fine. I had a really nice time while I was in Boston and now I'm even more excited about getting started!

On another note, I'm breaking up with my fiancé. It's a long story. I really don't want to get into it. But since I know that this relationship has a lot to do with how I feel right now, I'll tell you more next time I write.

I feel awful about this. Thank God for this project. Right now, it's the only thing I have going for me.

Reply from Michael

Hi Mandy,

I'm sorry to hear about your breakup. If you'd like to talk about it, please let me know.

For the time being, here are a few suggestions:

1. Go to an Al-Alon meeting. You could use some support right now and you should get a lot of it there.

2. Make an appointment with your doctor. Tell him about your participation in the project and that your trainer/therapist thinks you may have ADD. Ask him about the possibility of taking Wellbutrin (both to control your food cravings and to address your ADD). It's

---

MANDY'S UFOs

Insulin Instability

Attention Deficit Disorder (ADD)

Seasonal Affective Disorder (SAD)

"Askaphobia" (Fear of Asking for Help)

"Cantdoenza" (Self-Defeating Beliefs)

Premenstrual Dysphoric Disorder (PMDD)

Body Dysmorphic Disorder (BDD)

Energy Blocks/Reversals

"Heavy Baggage Syndrome" (Unresolved Emotional Issues)

Perfectionism

pretty clear that this is a problem for you, and that until you resolve it, you're apt to have trouble staying focused and following through on things, i.e., a diet or exercise program. While there are other options (besides Wellbutrin), given your history of depression, carbo-hydrate cravings, and (possibly) ADD, it may be the best route to take. Let's discuss.

Journal Entry #8

Hi Michael,
I just got home from work. I'm glad that I went because it got my mind off this whole relationship thing. It's amazing how many people are telling me that this breakup is for the best. We'll see . . .

Well, tonight at work I took a bite of this wonderful 8-inch choco-late chip cookie with caramel and chocolate sauce and nuts and ice cream and . . . okay stop me! Anyway, did I ever get hell for it! (My coworkers all know about this project.) My boss said, "You better tell Michael that you ate that!" And I said, "Wait, I swear, I don't start until Monday!" Nobody cared!

Anyway, I promise I will go to see my psychiatrist soon. Also the Al-Alon meetings are Monday nights at 7 P.M. I already looked into it.

I have a question: I like to work out in the morning. Do you recom-mend that I eat before or after my workout? So many people say so many different things! What do you think?

Reply from Michael

Hi Mandy,
If possible, have a light breakfast at least an hour before you work out. Some experts say that you'll burn more fat if you train on an empty stomach, but in my opinion, this is vastly exaggerated in terms of its benefit and isn't worth the loss of energy that you'll experience as a result.

Throughout the next twelve weeks, you'll be challenged to stay on course (you're bound to encounter people who will question what you do). Just do your best to stay focused and refer any questions to me. The last thing you need is anyone giving you questionable advice.

By the way, what prompted the decision (re: the breakup)? Was it something that we discussed?

Journal Entry #9

Hi Michael,

I can't say exactly what prompted the decision. When I called him from the airport, he started yelling at me about trivial events that happened before our relationship even started. I'm so tired of fighting with him. I'm tired of not being able to talk to him about what I do (or want to do) because I'm afraid he'll get mad. For example, going out with my friends, buying new shoes, going out to eat . . . even skipping class! I'm only twenty-two and sometimes I want to act like it!

Michael, two months ago we were planning this wonderful wedding and today I'm packing up his stuff. This is the hardest thing I've ever done. I've been crying all day wondering what I'm going to do. And now I'm going to have all these bills to take care of (everything was put in my name because he has bad credit). I can't break the lease and I can't just move to my sorority house because I have a dog. Nothing in the world would make me give her up! I can't even begin to explain the rest of my situation, it's just too complicated. Have you ever planned your future around something and had it crumble right before your eyes?

Well, I'll stop with my pity party and go find one of my sorority sisters to cry to. I just wonder why this is happening to me, especially now, as I begin this project. My life is a damn soap opera and a really bad one at that! I'll send you an E-mail about my first day of the program. Wish me luck!

Week 1—Journal Entry #10

Well, here I am back from my workout, having just finished lunch. I must say that it felt great to be back in the gym, although my time did consist of a lot of trial and error. I'd set up a machine, adjust the weight, adjust the seat, and then realize that the weight was too easy or the seat wasn't quite right. So I'd change the weight, hop off the machine, readjust it, and get back on. Taking a copy of my routine to the gym was very helpful. I know that next time will go much smoother because I'll be able to refer to the adjustments that I recorded in my log.

I adjusted quickly to moving more slowly, even though I've never trained that way before. At one point I did feel a little silly when the guy next to me pounded out ten reps for every one of my two. But I didn't let it affect me and I just kept right on going. Even though for some exercises I would only do six reps, I was delighted to finish my workout feeling like I'd worked up a good sweat. This rarely happened with my old way of training.

Now that I'm home I can really feel my muscles! Doing each stretch for thirty seconds also helped (instead of for the five or so seconds I'd do before). I was happy to see that my gym had all the machines listed for Cycle One except for three: the chest press, the abdominal crunch, and the lower-back extension. So I used comparable machines.

Even though my world often revolves around food, I've found that so far I haven't had any trouble following the plan. I have yet to feel hungry and I actually feel energized! Even "spunky"! I do, however, have to face the fact that finals are next week, bills are due, and my ex and I are finalizing our breakup today. I know I will be fine, though, because I *already* have more self-confidence! It's amazing what one day back in the gym can do! That, and a cute guy asked me to spot him on the bench press. Of course, I gladly offered my services!

MANDY

Weight, girth measurements, and body fat percentage, before:

Height: 5'3½"
Weight: 182 lbs.
Chest (bust): 41½"
Waist: 35½"
Hips: 43"
Upper thighs: 25¼" (L), 24¾" (R)
Calves: 16" (L), 16" (R)
Ankles: 8½" (L), 8½" (R)
Upper arms: 15" (L), 15" (R)
Forearms: 10½" (L), 11" (R)
Wrists: 6" (L), 6¼"(R)
Body fat: 32.5%

Week 1—Journal Entry #11

It's 5 P.M. and I have yet to exercise today, mainly because I retreated to my mom's house after my ex and I had a big fight. I didn't enjoy watching him move out, and since I no longer have a couch to sit on, I packed up the dog and went home to see my mommy.

It has been really hard to stick to "the plan" today, because there is absolutely no food here at my mom's house (that is, unless you consider "Hungry Man" TV dinners food). But I didn't see this listed on my plan, so I've steered clear! Watching TV hasn't made things any easier.

Because it's the holiday season, just about every channel has a show on where somebody is cooking up something tasty. For example, Rosie O'Donnell was making egg nog, which I love, and chocolate brownie sundaes! But somehow I've managed to stay on track, even with limited resources. For instance, breakfast was an egg white omelet with ham. But I can't tell you how good a pizza sounds right now! And I would love to have some egg nog!

Oh well, I'm off to the market for some chicken breasts and broccoli. I think I'll pick up some rye bread, too (if I don't get a carb fix soon I will surely die!).

I'm tired of struggling into my size 14 jeans. Now a size 8 . . . I could live with that!

Ten days later . . .

Hi Mandy,
I know it's a busy time of the year, but I'm concerned that I haven't heard from you. In fact, I've put the word out that you're MIA. Don't be surprised if you see your picture on the back of a milk carton!

Best wishes to you for a happy new year! This could be the best one yet!

Week 3—Journal Entry #12

Hi Michael,
Sorry I haven't written. I haven't had access to a computer until now. School is out for break and now that I'm single, I no longer have

a computer at home. I'm in Tekamah (Mom's house) and have been since before Christmas.

Being home for the holiday has really hindered my program because I don't have access to a gym or any equipment. But for the most part, I'm still eating better. I have lost some weight, but I'm not sure that it's really that noticeable.

I do notice that when I stick to the plan I feel great! I don't get cravings, I'm not severely hungry (like I used to be in the afternoon), and I no longer need a nap to make it through the day! The energy I have is just incredible! I also notice that after my workouts I have enough energy to go home and do other things. In the past I'd just go home and pass out.

I can't wait to start seeing more improvement. I just need to get back on my regular schedule and quit running all over the place. I can also tell that when I do miss a workout or have a bad day eating, physically I don't feel well. Mainly sluggish and tired. I really think you hit the nail on the head with regard to my diet! Plan B works great for me.

You'll be happy to hear that I've become really creative with veggies and spices. I never realized the world of fruits and vegetables could be so exciting (ha, ha)! Anyway, I'm starting the new year with no resolutions, just the motto "new year, new me." I'm excited about so many things. Many opportunities have opened up for me now that I'm "single."

I'm looking at an internship for this summer and I'm having fun thinking about the different possibilities I'll have after graduation (where I'll work, where I'll live, etc.). Whatever I want to do, I can! It's great! And this program will be the catalyst!

Week 4—Journal Entry #13

Hi Michael,

Well, I weighed myself on two different scales. One said 180 and the other said 174, so I'm now searching for a third scale.

For the first time in my life I feel that I'm doing this for myself. I no longer have anyone poking my sides, calling me fat, and telling me that I need to start exercising. I was also thinking . . . now that I'm single, I'm even *less* happy with the way I look. I feel self-conscious

> For the first time in my life I feel that I'm doing this for myself. I no longer have any-one poking my sides, calling me fat, and telling me that I need to start exercising.

> One minute I want some chips and salsa and the next minute I'll see a girl who is in great shape and think, "I need to cut back even more." One of my biggest prob-lems is comparing myself to other peo-ple. I know I shouldn't, but I do.

around guys. Especially guys I'm attracted to. Going into another relationship with this body is not an option!

Week 5—Journal Entry #14

Hi Michael,
My clothes are fitting looser this week, but it could be because they're stretched out. I saw my mom Saturday and asked her if I looked thinner. She said no. That wasn't very encouraging. But I'm not going to let it get me down! I'm determined not to let mental and environmental factors stand in my way. If anybody asks, by the way, this is the hardest thing I've ever done. Staying on track is very difficult, especially when I see all my friends eating pizza, drinking beer, etc. So I'm torn, because one minute I want some chips and salsa and the next minute I'll see a girl who is in great shape and think, "I need to cut back even more." One of my biggest problems is comparing myself to other people. I know I shouldn't, but I do.

Week 5—Journal Entry #15

Hi Michael,
Did I tell you I bought a scale? It was the one on which I weighed 180 (the last time I reported my weight via E-mail). I weighed myself about twenty minutes ago and I weigh (according to that scale) 175! Progress!

Did I mention that I have a date on Saturday? My friend and I are going on a dinner train to see a "who done it" murder mystery. It should be fun. For dinner I chose the blue-tipped shark. Is that on the list?

Anyway, I had to go shopping to find a dress to wear. I also bought a pair of jeans, which were actually a size 12! The last time I shopped for jeans I couldn't even button a size 12. What's cool is that it's the same style of jeans from the same store, so you can't chalk it up to differences in brand or style.

Well, with regard to your question about how I'm doing on Well-butrin, I feel wonderful! I'm so much more focused. And energized! My friends say I seem happier than I've been in a long time. So as far as my meds go, I'm doing very well. I feel so much better than I did, say, at the end of November.

Not much more to add today. All right, I'm off to the gym.

Week 5—Journal Entry #16

Hi Michael,

I apologize for missing the call last night. I was at Greg's house (my date from Saturday) and it completely slipped my mind. Per Cheryl's suggestion, though, I have been writing down ten positive things (about myself) every day!

And guess what? I now have a new computer! Very exciting! No more reasons to not write as often. And by the way, I'm feeling thinner!

Week 6—Journal Entry #17

It is such a gorgeous day. I can't wait to take Sadie out for a jog. It's also Friday! I don't think things could be any better! I've lost another pound (that makes seven total) and I was able to tighten my belt two more notches. This hasn't happened for years! You'll also be pleased to know that I've continued to write positive things about myself every day. It's a little embarrassing, though. I sound like that Stuart Smalley character (from *Saturday Night Live*). Anyway, here are a few examples:

- I'm a good singer
- I have a nice complexion
- I have cute feet
- My dog loves me
- I'm a fast typer
- I'm a good cook (even when it's low fat)
- I'm pleasant to be around
- People enjoy my company
- My teacher, Lila, says I am a beautiful woman

My friends and I are busy planning our trip to Vegas for spring break. Don't worry . . . I'll watch what I eat while I'm out there, but I won't have a gym to go to. We'll be walking a lot, so at least I'll be getting a little exercise. And hey, it's spring break! One week won't kill me, right? It will definitely be fun. And I'll get to see my grandpa again!

> 66
> You'll be pleased to know that I've continued to write positive things about myself every day. It's a little embarrassing, though. I sound like that Stuart Smalley character (from *Saturday Night Live*).
> 99

So things right now are great, and I'm happier than I've ever been! Well, gotta go cause I can't sit inside any longer. Happy Friday!

Week 7—Journal Entry #18

Hi Michael,

Well, I've been keeping up with Cheryl's homework assignment (writing down ten things that I like about myself every day). It's getting a little easier. Here are a few from last week:

- I have pretty eyes (a stranger even told me that out of the blue)
- I have cool jeans (another compliment from a random person)
- I'm approachable
- I have a nice smile
- I have straight teeth
- I'm a good swimmer
- I'm physically strong
- I'm a good role model
- I have nice hair
- I'm computer literate
- I did well on my test Monday
- I keep a neat and tidy home
- I shovel my own sidewalk
- I'm confident about my social skills
- People remember me (I make a lasting impression)

I know, some of these are pretty lame. Anyway, per your suggestion, I also got on the Internet and found a whole bunch of things to do in Vegas besides drink and gamble! Like:

- Go to the NASCAR Winston Cup
- See Blue Man Group
- Watch the pirate battle at Treasure Island
- Watch the volcano at the Mirage erupt
- See the fountains at Bellagio
- See the conservatory at Bellagio
- Go on a horseback ride in the Red Rocks
- Go to the top of the Eiffel Tower
- Go on a Black Canyon River raft tour

- Ride in a helicopter over the strip at night
- Play laser tag
- Rock climbing (indoors)
- Go to see the Tournament of Kings at Excalibur
- Roller coasters!

So yes, there are tons of things to do, and many of them are free or really cheap! Great for a college kid. Well, I'll wrap up for now, but I'll be sure to write later this week.

Week 7—Journal Entry #19

Well, I woke up today feeling pretty "down." I'm not sure why. But I just finished lifting weights and now I feel much better. It is nice out today so I might take Sadie for a walk, too.

I weighed myself this afternoon instead of in the morning. I weighed 171 (with clothes). So it will be interesting to see what I weigh tomorrow morning (when I usually weigh myself). If I'm below 170 pounds it will be the first time in years . . . that would be great! I'm noticing that my waist and thighs are getting smaller! But even though my arms look more defined, I think they're pretty much the same size. My lower abdomen is still an eyesore, and probably will be for a while, since it's where I keep most of my weight.

I had some baked tortilla chips on Tuesday afternoon (ate half the bag). Oops. I couldn't believe how awful I felt afterward! Very run down and tired. I even took an hour nap. It's amazing that eating the wrong kind of carbs can have that affect on me. When I stick to the diet, I consistently have a high level of energy. There's no question that it's the right plan for me.

I can tell the days are getting longer, not only because it stays lighter later in the day, but because the morning sun is shining in my room again! It's great to know that spring is on its way. After all, it will be shorts-wearing weather before we know it!

Week 8—Journal Entry #20

I'll tell you what . . . I am wiped out. I bought a pair of really nice rollerblades on Monday, and today I thought I would break them in. Thought I'd take my dog with me, too, but I soon discovered that the combination of me being a little rusty and her running around like a maniac wasn't a good one. So I dropped her off at home.

I decided to blade back and forth on the two blocks near my house. It's a quiet street, and I figured that if I wiped out, at least I wouldn't be too far from home (and could easily call an ambulance if necessary!). Well, after about fifteen minutes I was exhausted! Even in thirty-degree weather I was sweating buckets! Needless to say, I didn't do my usual twenty-five minutes (of cardio). But after I rest a bit I'll be strapping them back on for an afternoon skate. I'm happy about this because I've found something new to do that is both challenging and fun. It's amazing how a new exercise can make such a difference!

Week 8—Journal Entry #21

Well, I just checked out the website of the hotel I'll be staying at. I wanted to see if they had a fitness facility and they do! A large gym, a jogging track, and a year-round outdoor pool. I love to swim, too, so it'll be another fun way to get some cardiovascular exercise. It's nice to know I can keep up my weight training at this hotel because it's actually my favorite part of the program. It has really helped boost my confidence. And feeling strong makes me feel a lot safer, for example, in a parking lot at night, walking to my car.

Knowing that I'll have plenty of exercise options makes me even more excited about this trip. Vegas, here I come!

Reply from Michael

Hi Mandy,
That's great! I'm glad you found a good place to work out.
I'm happy to hear that you've been feeling so good lately! It's clear that the Wellbutrin is really helping you, increasingly more, in fact, as time progresses. And I think getting out in the sun more to exercise has helped you, too (with your SAD).
I'm happy to hear that you're enjoying your inline skates. And I'm relieved to hear that you didn't crash into a tree.
Have a great time in Vegas!

Hi Michael,

I really enjoyed our chat last night. It was nice to have a little pep talk before my trip.

Here are my current measurements:

Waist: 32½"
Chest: 39"
Hips: 39"

I don't remember what they were when we started, but all of my clothes are very loose. So something must be happening. Did I mention I bought a new belt? It's quite a bit shorter than my old ones. What fun!

Anyway, I need to get going. Thanks for sending the energy treatments!

Week 10—Journal Entry #23

Hi Michael,

Things are still going really well! People are starting to notice that I'm dropping weight and toning up. Now even people who don't know about the project are telling me how great I look. I ran into my old boss in the grocery store and she said she couldn't believe how much I've changed. Which is a big compliment coming from her (she is in great shape).

A few days ago Greg asked me if I'd lost more weight. I said, "Yes, why do you ask?" and he just smiled really big. This meant a lot to me because until then he hadn't seemed to notice. So the diet is going really well. I honestly didn't think I'd stick to it, but it makes me feel so much better that I can't even imagine going back to my old way of eating. I enjoy having a consistently high (and stable) energy level. I don't get hunger pains like I used to, either.

Now I'm confident that I won't go back to my former ways (once the project ends). Exercise isn't a task anymore—it's something I *want* to do!

Week 11—Journal Entry #24

Hi Michael,

I feel awful. I don't know if it's a cold or what, but I have no energy at all. When I get up in the morning I feel okay, but once I start doing things I feel like I want to crawl back into bed. I'm so tired. I took some over-the-counter stuff, but it made me dizzy and shaky. Last night, my ears were bothering me, too. Today I haven't taken anything (for the congestion), but I still feel horrible. If I still feel this bad tomorrow I'll make an appointment with the campus doctor.

So this week I haven't worked out at all, which really stinks because my photo shoot is in nine days! I haven't even made it to class this week! Talk about bad timing . . .

Reply from Michael

It sounds like you may have a sinus infection. Go to your doctor ASAP (you may need an antibiotic). Take care of yourself!

Week 12—Journal Entry #25

Hi Michael,

I feel much better today! You were right, it was a sinus infection, and the antibiotic kicked in fast. So I even did a little exercise today. I'll give it another day or so before I do anything too strenuous.

Since this will probably be my last journal entry, here are some general thoughts:

This project has been a lifesaver. I really learned a lot. The diet (Plan B) turned out to be the perfect thing for me. I'm clearly insulin sensitive and I was eating too many carbs. I was put on a plan to address this and it really did the job! My energy level increased a lot and I stopped having energy swings. Before I started this program, I napped every day at 3 P.M. I was putting things off all the time because I was always feeling so tired. Now I don't need to nap at all. I have energy all day!

I've also been sleeping much better and have stopped craving fattening things. Even around my cycle, I crave sweets much less than before. And I no longer feel so hungry (I used to be snacking all the

331 ■
Mandy

time!). Being on Wellbutrin may have helped to reduce my cravings, too. Most importantly, though, it helped me to focus and be more clear. Learning that I had ADD was critical to my success.

Changing my eating habits wasn't as hard as I thought it would be. Anytime I went off the diet, I could really tell the difference. I'd be sluggish, bloated, and tired. But as soon as I'd start eating healthy again, I would feel a lot better, quick.

At first, when I was taught how to exercise slowly and with more control, I honestly thought that training this way would take me a lot more time. It turned out *not* to be true. What a difference it makes! Now I spend less time in the gym (doing fewer reps and sets) and no longer feel "stuck" (unable to make more progress). Once I get used to a workout, I simply go to the next cycle, which is always a little more challenging (and prevents me from getting bored). My muscles just keep getting stronger and are much more shapely and toned. Also, when I move slowly, I can really feel the "burn," which I love because it shows how much my muscles are being worked.

MANDY

Weight, girth measurements, and body fat percentage, after 12 weeks*:

Height: 5'3½"
Weight: 167 lbs. (−15 lbs.)
Chest (bust): 40½" (−1")
Waist: 32½" (−3")
Hips: 41½" (−1½")
Upper thighs: 24¼" (L), 24" (R) (−1", −¾")
Calves: 15¼" (L), 15¼" (R) (−¾", −¾")
Ankles: 8¼" (L), 8¼" (R) (−¼", −¼")
Upper arms: 13½" (L), 13¾" (R) (−1½", −1¼")
Forearms: 10" (L), 10¼" (R) (−½", −¾")
Wrists: 5¾" (L), 6" (R) (−¼", −¼")
Total inches lost: 13¾"
Body-fat: 26% (−6.5%)

*Seven weeks total in training.

Because I'm a senior in college, I took this on at a challenging time. The hardest thing for me was feeling the need to socialize. When you're in college, if you want to be where the action is, the place to go on a Thursday, Friday, or Saturday night is, of course, the bar. I'm a very social person and I love to hang out with my friends. And so there were times that I'd go to a bar and eat pizza at 2 A.M. There were also times that I didn't drink, but it really wasn't much fun. I really had to be disciplined in order to stay away.

Spring break was another challenge. I went to Vegas a couple of times, and if it wasn't for some strategic preplanning (Michael had me make a list of "healthy" things I could do), I might not have stayed on course.

Now that I'm single, I'm actually more motivated to exercise (being more confident about my body helps me feel less insecure). Thankfully, this project has really helped me in that regard. I'm also starting to focus on things I *like* about myself (instead of things I dislike). This is a major change.

As I think about what I've been through, I'm amazed that I've done so well. Considering that I broke up with my fiancé, was in my last semester in school, went away for spring break (twice), got sick a few times, and was tempted every day at school by pizza, junk food, and beer, I'd have to say that I've succeeded—on a number of different levels. And this is only the beginning! I've got so much to look forward to!

Thank you for all of your help!
Mandy

CHAPTER FOURTEEN

NINA

I'm tired of people thinking of me as the big frumpy girl next door.

Nina

Age: 33
Height: 5'6"
Weight: 165 lbs.
Occupation: Administrative Assistant,
   Stanford University School of Medicine

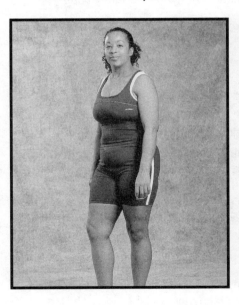 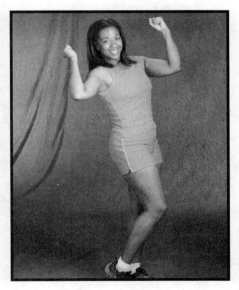

Excerpt from letter:

*Only a year ago, I weighed 60 pounds more than I do now. Six years ago,
I actually weighed 280 pounds. I'm proud of myself for coming so far,
but now I feel like I'm stuck. I seem to be making less progress. I want to
lose 30 pounds more.*

Journal Entry #1

Today feels like the beginning of a dream. I'm very excited about this project and looking forward to the next few months.

Whoever said "the possibilities are endless" wasn't kidding! It's one of my favorite sayings (the other being "take the smart risk").

Journal Entry #2

I met with my brother Jamie today. I enjoyed spending time with him. We talked a lot about how I was able to finally start losing weight. He was wondering how I did it (and why I had gained so much in the past). I told him that I changed my view of eating and working out. In the past, I saw it as something that had to be "managed" (which caused me stress). Now, I see it as something that is a natural part of my life. In other words, I changed my mind and my body followed suit.

Journal Entry #3

I worked at the Gap today and it was crazy, to say the least. I forgot to bring an apple with me (or a piece of fruit) for a snack, so I ended up at McDonald's, where I just had to have some fries! This is one of the reasons that I hate spending time at the mall . . . they don't have too many places where you can get a healthy snack!

When I got home, for dinner, I had a piece of carrot cake. I know . . . shame on me, but I was just too tired to cook!

Journal Entry #4

I wore my black suit to work today and I must say, it looked great! But I need to expand my wardrobe (the more weight I lose, the less my clothes fit). It seems like I have to go shopping for something new to wear each week!

I'm looking forward to my trip to Boston! Tonight I will read your book . . .

Journal Entry #5

I am completely frustrated with my wardrobe! But I guess I shouldn't be. After all, I'm the one who wanted to lose weight! One day, I will shop till I drop!

Mental note . . . a menstrual cycle is not a free pass to eat junk food and sweets! Hello? No more sweets for the rest of the week!

Journal Entry #6

I'm feeling a little down today. Often at this time of year I think of the loved ones that I've lost. Of course, it makes me very sad. I feel very much alone.

Today I thank God for my brothers, David, Jamie, and Xavier, my sister-in-law Lily, my beautiful nephew Yamato, and gorgeous niece Sakura (a spitting image of my mother, who every day is sorely missed).

Journal Entry #7

I read something in Michael's book today that really hit close to home: my fear of looking "too good" (by losing weight) and attracting men. When I was eleven years old, I started modeling in a road show. I think this was much too young for me to be doing such a thing. All the attention I got felt weird and really creeped me out. I was scared that, like my mother, I would attract the wrong kind of man.

My mother had bad luck when it came to choosing and dating men. I didn't want to repeat her mistakes and have kids at such a young age. I think I turned to food as a way to shield myself from men . . .

Journal Entry #8

I decided this morning that I would weigh myself just once a week. When I weigh myself more often than this, I tend to fight with myself.

It's amazing how you can actually think you're looking pretty good, but then see yourself in a swimsuit and completely be freaked out. At least my waist looked smaller and my arms were more defined. And my face is a good deal slimmer than it has been in a long time.

> " I read something in Michael's book today that really hit close to home: my fear of looking "too good" (by losing weight) and attracting men. "

Journal Entry #9

I think I may suffer from SAD. I don't like the winter at all. It's hard for me to get out of bed and I have more cravings for sweets. Fortunately, the past two winters haven't been as bad.

Journal Entry #10

I'm almost finished with Michael's book. It has made me question some things. He refers a great deal to "the Zone" in his book (a plan I'm not sure that I like). I'm anxious to hear what he wants me to do (compared to what I do now).

Journal Entry #11

Hi Michael,
Just wanted to say sayonara before I leave for Okinawa. I also wanted to let you know that I finished reading your book. Here are what (I think) are some of my primary UFOs:

- Obsession with burning calories
- Improper food combining
- PMS
- Suppressed emotional conflicts
- Failure to vary training mode
- Exercise addiction

I can't wait to take your UFO test to see what else it reveals. I look forward to seeing you soon!

Journal Entry #12

Hi Michael,
I'm back and all is well. It was great meeting you! I look forward to working with you and all of the other folks on your team. It's been two days since I last had sweets, and I'm already feeling great!

Thank you for all of your help and advice (I look forward to getting more!). This week is starting off splendidly—thank you, once again!

Hi Nina,

Glad to hear that you made it back . . . happy, safe, and sound. It was really great to meet you. Now get ready for twelve great weeks!

You'll be happy to hear that I've scored your UFO test (please see below). Here are some thoughts and observations based on what it revealed:

First, we need to address the way that you've been combining foods. In general, avoid eating vegetables at the same time that you eat fruit. Also avoid eating starchy carbs with any high-protein foods. Starchy carbs include cereal, rice, potatoes, pasta, and bread. High-protein foods include red meat, most nuts, soy, fish, and eggs. If you do combine these foods, you won't absorb nutrients very well, and you may have digestive problems, for example, heartburn and gas. Fortunately, food combining has been addressed somewhat by Plan B.

Your "insulin instability" should be corrected with Plan B, but as discussed, we may also have to address a problem with yeast. This will become much clearer over the course of the next few weeks.

NINA

Weight, girth measurements, and body fat percentage, before:

Height: 5'6"
Weight: 165 lbs.
Chest (bust): 40½"
Waist: 31¾"
Hips: 43½"
Upper thighs: 24½" (L), 24½" (R)
Calves: 15" (L), 15" (R)
Ankles: 8¼" (L), 8¼" (R)
Upper arms: 11½" (L), 11½" (R)
Forearms: 9½" (L), 9½" (R)
Wrists: 6" (L), 6" (R)
Body fat: 31.5%

Regarding ADD, let's tackle the first seven UFOs first. Once you alter your diet and learn how to manage your PMS, you may become much more focused and have less trouble finishing tasks.

Regarding your PMS issues, there's a good chance that the diet will help. Use your journal entries to keep a record of how you feel. We may want to try some supplements and have you talk to Tracy Gaudet.

And last but not least, I hope that you'll learn to get better at asking for help! I know that your faith is very strong, so "ask and ye shall receive!" We'll discuss this in greater detail, I'm sure, the next time that we speak.

That's about it for now. I'm very excited to hear how you do! Let's be sure to talk real soon, and have a great first week!

Week 1—Journal Entry #13

Day four has started out great! Other than cocoa this morning, I've had no sweets for four days. Four days has been the longest that I think I've *ever* gone!

My menstrual cycle starts this week (along with my cravings for sweets). I always gain 2 or 3 pounds each month—the same 2 or 3 that I lose!

Plan B (the Zone) is like what I'm doing already, so it should be fine. But now it's almost 5 P.M. and I'm not feeling satisfied. This is probably due to the fact that I always was "sneaking" sweets—a

---

NINA'S UFOs

Premenstrual Dysphoric Disorder (PMDD)
Insulin Instability
Seasonal Allergies
Candidiasis
Improper Food Combining
Perfectionism
Exercise Addiction
Attention Deficit Disorder (ADD)
Weak Boundaries
"Askaphobia" (Fear of Asking for Help)

Power Bar, a granola bar, anything I could find. I guess this will be a challenge, but it's one I feel ready to face.

Reply from Michael

Nina, just so you know, that plan that you're on is not "the Zone." On this plan, you're required to have more low-glycemic carbs (50 percent of your intake, rather than 40, like the Zone).

Week 1—Journal Entry #14

It's still very cold outside (to me) and I love eating warm, sweet foods. I guess that's why I always gain weight every year during the winter months.

I could really feel yesterday's workout, particularly in my legs (the chest and arm exercises didn't seem to be as intense). While doing each exercise slowly, my muscles were feeling more stressed (compared to when I would use more weight and do each exercise fast).

Reply from Michael

Hi Nina,
If now your workout seems easy to you, remember, it's just the first week! You're only getting your feet wet and getting used to moving slowly. Your workout will quickly become more intense, so enjoy "the break" while you can!

> ❝
> My menstrual cycle starts this week (along with my cravings for sweets). I always gain 2 or 3 pounds each month —the same 2 or 3 that I lose!
> ❞

Week 2—Journal Entry #15

Great to hear from you, Michael—thanks so much for setting me straight. I'd like to move on to Cycle 2, but maybe I'm jumping the gun. Perhaps it is the perfectionist and/or overtrainer in me?

Talk to you later tonight!

Week 2—Journal Entry #16

Hi Michael,
I enjoyed the teleclass yesterday and liked all the things that you said. I've been having fun with this project so far and have already learned a lot.

On Sunday, my friend will be taping me while I'm training at the gym. I'll send you the tape as soon as I can and wait for your response.

Week 2—Journal Entry #17

I actually went to a movie today and didn't eat any sweets! I used to see two or three movies a week, eating popcorn and candy each time. Now I can see how it all added up and kept me from losing weight.

I raised my weights a little today (it was hard to finish ten reps). And although I was moving much slower, I actually spent *less* time in the gym! I think it's because I no longer have to do as many sets.

Week 2—Journal Entry #18

Today's good news is that I feel much fuller after I eat. I'm also not nearly as hungry and have more energy during the day. This plan seems to be about "balance"—eating the right combination of foods. Basically, I'm feeling satisfied (and happy to tell my friends!).

Reply from Michael

Hi Nina,

I received your fax—thanks for sending! A couple of things:

- It seems that you usually end your sets as soon as you do ten reps. If this is the case, you're probably not reaching failure (total fatigue). From now on, try to get to this point on each exercise (with good form).
- You're doing pretty well calorie-wise, but your vegetable servings are low. Try to be more mindful of this whenever you plan your meals.
- Instead of doing lots of sets and reps to train your abs, I'd like you to stick to the program, i.e., work harder and do fewer sets. If you're able to do twelve reps or more with strict, controlled technique, I suggest that you hold a weight, either under your chin or behind your head (don't hold the weight behind your head if it puts too much strain on your neck). It's more important to use more weight than it is to do lots of reps!

Today's good news is that I feel much fuller after I eat. I'm also not nearly as hungry and have more energy during the day. This plan seems to be about "balance"— eating the right combinations of foods.

• I'm glad to hear that your workout isn't taking as long to do. On this program, you'll work twice as hard in half the amount of time! This will be more apparent when you progress to Cycle 3.

Week 2—Journal Entry #19

I really love getting advice from you. I'll do what you recommend!

And I know . . . I should eat more vegetables, so I'll work on that tonight. I'm going to have tomato soup (does that count as a vegetable, too?).

Week 3—Journal Entry #20

It now has become second nature to eat the right foods and stick to my plan. In fact, I no longer need to look at the plan to know what to do!

I ate some fruit after dinner and my stomach paid the price. I forgot that I had vegetables, and they don't sit well with fruit!

Week 3—Journal Entry #21

I can already see the results of going to failure and moving slowly. On Thursday, I'm looking forward to beginning Cycle 3.

Week 3—Journal Entry #22

I weighed myself today and was pleased to see that I've lost 4 pounds! Less than ten weeks to go, and I already look more defined. I'm starting to see the muscles in my shoulders, stomach, and back. And my legs are looking slimmer, not to mention my upper arms!

This week I plan to deal with some UFOs that I've yet to address. Oddly enough, I think that some have already worked themselves out!

Week 4—Journal Entry #23

The 12th day of the month is often one that makes me sad. My mother was born on the 12th of July, and I'm still mourning her loss. I once heard someone say that death is great for the person who dies, and only bad for the loved ones who that person leaves behind. Based on my experience, I believe that this is true.

The nutritional plan that I am on has helped me in many ways. For example, this month, I wasn't bothered as much by PMS. I had a few cramps on the first day, but not nearly as bad as before. I even took less Advil and still had a lot less pain. And while in the past, I took flaxseed oil and calcium, which did help, it never really did anything to reduce the pain in my back. But now I can say, without question, that eating this way has really helped.

The best thing about this plan is that it helps with my PMS, and helps me feel more energized, full, and satisfied after meals.

Week 4—Journal Entry #24

I was just telling some coworkers that my crush is in town this week! I said that I wanted to get dolled up and take his breath away. How strange for you to challenge me to do the very same thing!

I'm disappointed, though, that I haven't lost anything in three days. It's bumming me out that my weight is the same, even though I've given up sweets.

Week 4—Journal Entry #25

Well . . . the scale hasn't moved, but my clothes get baggier every day. And believe it or not, I tightened my belt another notch today! Coolness!

Week 4—Journal Entry #26

Hey, I took your challenge and in a way, it was a success. I didn't get to impress my crush, but I did something else instead. A coworker and I went out for a drink and hung out for a while at a bar. I wore a black, body-conscious dress and thought that I looked pretty good. I even caught the attention of a waiter who seemed pretty nice, but I didn't know how to move forward so I just got up and left. Oh well, I have some learning to do. I'll have to do better next time!

Week 5—Journal Entry #27

Today I went hiking near Stanford on a popular trail called "the Dish." The last time I did this trail my muscles were sore for two or three days! But this time around, it surprised me that I didn't get sore at all.

I've also been doing some yoga and I think this is helping me, too. Now that I'm stronger, I'm holding my poses up to a minute or more!

I had a slice of pumpkin bread the other day at work. Less than an hour later, I found myself fighting to stay awake. I really don't like when I feel that way, so I won't let it happen again!

It has been almost three weeks since I've had cookies, donuts, or cake. I can't wait to get to the point where I'm not always craving sweets!

Week 6—Journal Entry #28

During tonight's teleclass, Cheryl discussed the power of negative thoughts. While I make a conscious effort to be positive all the time, I was able to see that there are times when this is hard to do. What she said reminded me of a book I've started to read. It's called *Conversations with God* and the author is Neale Donald Walsch.

Week 6—Journal Entry #29

Hi Michael,
Sorry I missed your call, but in a way, I'm glad I did. This week was not very good for me—I strayed quite a bit from "the plan." Burgers, fries, a chocolate shake, and sweets four days in a row!

Week 6—Journal Entry #30

Today is the day that my cycle starts. But things have been better this month. I've had very little bloating and almost no back pain at all! I think that eating better (and taking supplements) really has helped.

Week 7—Journal Entry #31

Believe it or not, I haven't weighed myself in about two weeks. I am letting go of my hang-ups and paying attention to how I feel. Speaking of which, it feels great to have a toned stomach and thinner thighs!

Week 7—Journal Entry #32

Right at this moment, I'm eating one of my latest favorite treats.
A Luna peanut butter bar with chocolate and lots of nuts.
They're great to take to the movies, since there's not much else
I can eat. Pretzels are good, and popcorn is, too, but these foods
aren't allowed on my plan.

I'm still on my menstrual cycle, but it should be over soon. I think
that is why my weight has increased a bit (to 156).

Reply from Michael

Hi Nina,
I took a look at your workout log, and your reps are much too high!
Select a weight that makes you "fail" somewhere between 6–10 reps
(8–12 on abs and calves). If you can't do at least six reps with perfect form, then lower the weight. If you're able to do at least ten
reps, then you should increase the weight.

Also, I hate to tell you this, but no Luna bars on Plan C! Most nuts
are fine for a snack now and then, but peanuts are not allowed. Sorry!

Week 7—Journal Entry #33

I talked to Michael last night and once again, he set me straight.
I knew that I had it coming with all that cake I had last week. He also
said that I need to go to failure on each set. I guess he could tell
(since my reps were the same on each set) that I stop short! I also
need to remember to use more weight whenever I can.

Week 7—Journal Entry #34

My friend and I went dancing tonight and really had a blast. Men love
to hold up the walls and sip their drinks and check women out, but
none of them have the guts, it seems, to ask a lady to dance!

Week 8—Journal Entry #35

I'm feeling pretty good today. My stomach is getting flat. And now I
can only pinch an inch instead of four or five. My legs are looking lean
and feeling strong, as is my back!

> 66
>
> This week was not
> very good for me—
> I strayed quite a bit
> from "the plan." Burg-
> ers, fries, a chocolate
> shake, and sweets
> four days in a row!
>
> 99

Week 8—Journal Entry #36

Monday was a tough day for me. I said good-bye to a friend and remembered saying good-bye to my mom. I miss her very much. I know her spirit and soul are far better off where she is now, but I miss her kindness and warmth, as well as her smile and funny laugh.

Week 8—Journal Entry #37

I feel like I should be losing more weight (I'm still at 155). I wanted to be 140 pounds for the after shoot. I know I should be thankful that I've lost as much as I have, but I seem to be getting impatient now that I don't have many weeks left.

Week 9—Journal Entry #38

Tonight I'm going to The Cheesecake Factory. And yes, I'm going to have some cheesecake. I think the last time I had any was at our office Halloween party. I am long overdue!

Yesterday I wasn't happy, but I feel much better today. I sent recent photos to some of my friends, and their compliments picked me up. It's easy for me to forget sometimes, but I really have come a long way.

I heard my crush say (on the radio) that he's seeking the perfect girl. Well, if he's truly the one for me (and my gut tells me that he is), then I guess I'll just have to hope that I am perfect in his eyes . . .

Week 9—Journal Entry #39

Today I went shopping at the mall and discovered that I'm a size 8! I would never have thought it was possible back when I was a size 24!

Week 10—Journal Entry #40

Today I weigh 153 and I look great (if I say so myself!). My black pants are loose all over—even around my hips and thighs. Who would have ever thunk it back when I started (at week 1)?

I don't think (as an adult) I've ever weighed less than 175. In college, I kept gaining weight no matter what type of workout I did. I think it was mostly due to all the soda that I would drink. Even though I ran a lot and often worked out with weights, I didn't realize then how important it is to eat the right food.

Week 10—Journal Entry #41

It has been almost two weeks since I was switched from Plan B to Plan C. But although I have lost 2 pounds, I'm not really sure if it's due to the change.

My workouts are going well now that I've been lifting heavier weights. My back is shaping up beautifully, and my legs and abs are, too!

Week 10—Journal Entry #42

It's the week before my cycle and I'm actually *losing* weight! I think the B_6 and magnesium are helping me out a lot (thanks to Tracy Gaudet for her advice on last month's call). It's amazing how much my mood has improved. And I haven't been craving sweets!

Week 10—Journal Entry #43

This week has been a good one (I haven't suffered from PMS!). I guess the B_6 and magnesium are exactly what I need. I haven't had any back pain, and for the most part, minimal cramps. It's hard to believe that these supplements work so well for PMS. The calcium that I've been taking seems to be helping me out as well. And to this point, I haven't gained my usual 2 or 3 pounds!

The light therapy is okay, but I'm not really sure it has helped that much. Granted, I haven't been doing it much (I haven't had any time!).

Week 11—Journal Entry #44

I had a nice workout yesterday. I worked hard on my back and legs. Before, when I used to move faster, I really didn't feel much of a burn. But now I can see a big difference as a result of slowing down. I was always afraid to train my legs (I was worried that they would "bulk up"). But now, not only are they more toned, they're quite a bit slimmer, too!

> **"**
> Today I went shopping at the mall and discovered that I'm a size 8! I would never have thought it was possible back when I was a size 24!
> **"**

Week 11—Journal Entry #45

I'm hoping that by this summer, I'll be 135 pounds. But I'm in no rush to get there because I'm really enjoying the ride!

Week 11—Journal Entry #46

The teleclass was great last night, but it took me by surprise. When Debbie Ford asked what my "story" was, it triggered all kinds of stuff. I thought about how my past reflects the way I feel today. I remembered a lot of what happened back when I was eleven years old. Molestation, pregnancy, alcohol, drugs, abandonment, and abuse. I didn't "directly" experience *all* of this, but it's still a lot!

Week 11—Journal Entry #47

Today is a special day because I have lost another pound! Now I am 1 pound shy of being 150 pounds. I feel like I've spent the last two weeks or so around 155. So being able to get to this point seems almost too good to be true!

> **"**
> Now I can see a big difference as a result of slowing down. I was always afraid to train my legs (I was worried that they would "bulk up"). But not only are my legs more toned, they're quite a bit slimmer, too!
> **"**

NINA

Weight, girth measurements, and body fat percentage, after 12 weeks:

Height: 5'6"
Weight: 151 lbs. (−14 lbs.)
Chest (bust): 38" (−2½")
Waist: 28¾" (−3")
Hips: 40¼" (−3¼")
Upper thighs: 23¼") (L), 23¼" (R) (−1¼", −1¼")
Calves: 14¼" (L), 14¼" (R) (−¾", −¾")
Ankles: 8¼" (L), 8¼" (R) (no change)
Upper arms: 11" (L), 11" (R) (−½", −½")
Forearms: 9¼" (L), 9¼" (R) (−¼", −¼")
Wrists: 5¾" (L), 5¾" (R) (−¼", −¼")
Total inches lost: 14¾"
Body fat: 23% (−8.5%)

> **"**
> It's the week before my cycle and I'm actually *losing* weight! I think the B_6 and magnesium are helping me out a lot (thanks to Tracy Gaudet for her advice on last month's call).
> **"**

Week 11—Journal Entry #48

I'm eating more fruit and vegetables now, and the weight is coming right off. Only one week to go, and I am feeling like a champ!

Week 12—Journal Entry #49

Well, I've lost about 15 pounds and today I'm feeling great! I feel comfortable in my swimsuit and I like the way I look. I like my muscular legs, small waist, toned back, and well-defined arms.

Week 12—Journal Entry #50

What an amazing twelve weeks it has been! I feel like I've learned so much! At first, I learned how my thoughts affect how my body responds to stress. I lost 4 pounds (in only two weeks) and seemed to be right on track. Then, we discovered that one of my UFOs was PMS. To address it, I used B_6, magnesium, calcium, and bright light.

I have really enjoyed the classes, both with Cheryl and Debbie Ford. I've gained a lot of insight about myself from their books, as well. I now see why I use food to comfort myself (because of my past).

It took twelve weeks for me to see that I actually strayed from "the plan." I thought I had memorized it, but evidently, I was wrong! But even though I wasn't perfect, I experienced great success. For this, I am very thankful. I can't wait for the *next* twelve weeks!

> "
> It took twelve weeks for me to see that I actually strayed from "the plan." I thought I had memorized it, but evidently, I was wrong.
> "

ABOUT THE AUTHOR

Michael Gerrish, M.S., is the author of *When Working Out Isn't Working Out: A Mind-Body Guide to Conquering Unidentified Fitness Obstacles* (St. Martin's Press, 1999). He is also the host and creator of exerciseplus.com. Formerly a conditioning consultant for the Boston Red Sox and Boston Bruins, Michael is currently a fitness consultant, psychotherapist, and certified thought field therapist.

Michael, who has a B.S. in physical education/commercial recreation, an M.S. in counseling psychology, and a Level 2 Certification in thought field therapy, received his graduate and undergraduate degrees from Springfield College, in Springfield, Massachusetts.

Michael's work has been featured in *Fitness, Real Simple, Self, Mademoiselle, Oxygen, Muscle Media, Women's Day, Investor's Business Daily, Cosmopolitan, American Fitness, Muscle and Fitness,* the *Boston Globe,* the *New York Times,* the *Columbus Dispatch*, the *Denver Post*, the One Spirit Book Club, and many other publications and popular websites. He lives in Massachusetts with his wife, Cheryl Richardson, author of three *New York Times* best-selling books.

To contact Michael:

Michael Gerrish
P.O. Box 13
Newburyport, MA 01950
E-mail: michael@exerciseplus.com

To subscribe to a free newsletter or join a fitness makeover group, visit Michael's website at www.exerciseplus.com.

To contact Ginger Burr (image consultant):

Website: www.totalimageconsultants.com
Tel: 617-625-5225; 800-380-8726
Fax: 617-629-3939

To subscribe to Cheryl Richardson's free newsletter or join a life makeover group, visit her website at www.cherylrichardson.com.

INDEX